American Medical Association

Physicians dedicated to the health of America

Physician Practice Management Companies:
What You Need To Know

P. John Seward, MD, AMA Executive Vice President

Kirk B. Johnson, JD, AMA General Counsel and Group Vice President
for Health Policy Advocacy

Denise C. Andresen, JD, AMA Assistant General Counsel

American Medical Association Project Team

Helen Jameson, JD, Senior Attorney

Jill F. Blim, Private Sector Advocacy Team

Thomas Sharpe, Senior Acquisitions Editor, Physician Practice Products

Jean Roberts, Senior Editor

Selby Toporek, Senior Marketing Services Coordinator

Voni Giambrone, Marketing Manager

Physician Practice Management Companies: What You Need to Know

© Copyright 1997 American Medical Association. Printed in the USA

http://www.ama-assn.org

Additional copies of this publication may be obtained by contacting the
American Medical Association at 800 621-8335.

Disclaimer

This book is published by the American Medical Association for
educational purposes only. It is intended solely to provide general
information on affiliation with a physician practice management company
to assist physicians who may be contemplating such an endeavor. It is not
intended to constitute legal advice and should not be relied on as a source
of legal advice. If legal advice is desired or needed, a licensed attorney
should be consulted.

ISBN: 0-89970-857-9
OP 316696

BP38: 97-349:3M:7/97

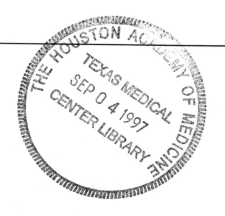

Table of Contents

Preface

This book is about physician practice management companies, or PPMCs — entities that were nonexistent a mere decade ago. PPMCs emerged in the late 1980s as a response to the rapid evolution of managed care and the increasing consolidation of physician practices. Today, approximately 5% of active US physicians are affiliated with PPMCs. By 2000, that number is expected to rise to 14%, indicating that more and more physicians are opting to affiliate with a PPMC as a way of strengthening their position in the marketplace. The stated goal of PPMCs is to offer physicians professional management expertise, to provide practices with capital for clinic expansion, and to handle the increasing complexities of group practice operations. The purpose of this book is to assist physicians and physician groups who are contemplating an affiliation make an informed and strategic decision.

It is important to note at the outset that practice management company affiliation is just one of many strategic options available to physician groups seeking to strengthen their position in the marketplace. While affiliation may be appropriate for some groups, it may not be for others. In this book we try to provide you with a balanced view of PPMCs, considering both the advantages and disadvantages associated with PPMC affiliation.

In the first chapter of this book you will be introduced to the market dynamics that currently exist in the health care environment and the ways physicians have chosen to respond to the changes that are taking place. Next you will be provided with an overview of the potential advantages and disadvantages of affiliating with a PPMC. In the third chapter we explore the organizational design of PPMCs and discuss the types of groups most often pursued by PPMCs for affiliation. Along with this discussion we present various checklists that will assist you in evaluating a PPMC as a strategic partner. The fourth chapter of this book is devoted to the techniques used by PPMCs in acquiring physician practices and to an examination of the growth trends in the PPMC industry. The final chapter offers a snapshot of the relationship between Wall Street and PPMCs. The appendices at the back of this book include descriptions of some existing public and private PPMCs and a review of the activities of these groups in the recent past.

Throughout our discussions you may encounter financial and accounting terms or expressions that may or may not be familiar to you, such as EBIT, price-to-earnings ratios, and discounted cash flow analysis. Whenever possible we have tried to explain financial concepts in terms that any person, regardless of their business background, can understand intuitively. The goal of this book is to make you an informed decision-maker, not an expert in finance.

The American Medical Association has published this book to offer physicans general information on PPMC affiliation and to assist them in making strategic choices. As is always the case, the reader should not rely on this book as legal or professional advice. If you are ready to proceed on a course of action, you should seek the assistance of a qualified attorney or business advisor.

Acknowledgments

The American Medical Association gratefully acknowledges the contribution of the following individuals in completing this publication.

Douglas Townsend and Jill Frew of Townsend Frew & Co.

Helen Jameson, JD, and Jill Blim of the Office of the General Counsel, Health Law Division, American Medical Association, who directed the content and edited the manuscript for this publication.

Douglas Hough, PhD, Argus·Arista Associates (Fairfax, VA), who allowed us to adapt material for use in Chapter 1: Strategic Options in a Changing Health Care Marketplace.

Norman Chenven, MD, of the Austin Regional Clinic (Durham, NC), who reviewed the manuscript and provided the editors with valuable comments and suggestions.

1 Strategic Options in a Changing Health Care Marketplace

This chapter will provide you with an understanding of the current market dynamics in the health care environment and will introduce you to two of the many strategic options that are available to medical practices as they struggle to remain competitive in the marketplace: expanding the practice independently and selling to a strategic partner. We will then begin to explore the nature of physician practice management companies (PPMCs) and offer some thoughts about how to best approach this unique strategic alternative.

The Changing Health Care Marketplace

The health care marketplace of today is different from that of 30 years ago when solo practitioners thrived and most physicians were paid on a fee-for-service basis. The advent of managed care has dramatically changed this landscape.

Managed care was an outgrowth of skyrocketing health care costs. As early as the 1970s, purchasers of health care began pushing for cost containment, leading to the development of managed care organizations and the passage of federal legislation encouraging the establishment of health maintenance organizations (HMOs). At least one HMO, Kaiser Permanente, has existed since the 1940s.

The level of managed care penetration in the United States has increased dramatically since the 1980s and is expected to continue growing. In 1980, 4% of the U.S. population was enrolled in an HMO. By 1995, that percentage had grown to about 22%, and it is expected to reach 47% by the year 2002. This growth in managed care has led to the consolidation of physician practices and also to the emergence of PPMCs.

Physician receipts currently account for $246 billion, or 23% of the market, and physicians influence over $900 billion, or 86% of health care expenditures, through their decisions. Consequently, with the advent of managed care, health plans have sought to contain the cost of providing medical care by introducing discounted fee-for-service and capitated payment arrangements with physicians. Managed care organizations now require physicians to demonstrate "efficiency" in their practices. These arrangements and requirements can place many physician practices, particularly solo and small group practices, at a disadvantage because they do not have the appropriate infrastructure.

In markets with high managed care penetration, operation of solo practices is especially difficult, and many physicians have responded by either consolidating their practices with others or moving to another market. In markets with relatively low managed care penetration, physicians have more opportunity to take the initiative and develop strategies to stay in the driver's seat and maintain income levels. Nevertheless, even in markets with lower managed care penetration, a medical practice must overcome barriers in order to succeed.

Potential Barriers to Success in Managed Care

Lack of Capital

Succeeding in managed care often requires an infusion of capital that is beyond the reach of many physicians and physician groups. For example, health care purchasers increasingly demand that providers demonstrate that they provide high-quality, cost-effective care. Consequently, physicians must purchase information systems that supply the necessary cost and quality data required by payers under capitated and discounted fee-for-service arrangements. Also, physicians often need more administrative staff to evaluate the insurance risk of accepting managed care contracts, and the practice may need to acquire additional primary care physicians. The capital needed to build this managed care infrastructure can exceed $3 million for a clinic with 20 physicians.

Lack of Network

Some physicians and physician groups may not enjoy a competitive position with managed care companies because they lack formal ties with other more diverse or complementary physician groups. This limits their ability to offer coordinated care across several specialties, as well as their ability to control costs through group purchasing economies.

By broadening their network and becoming associated with other physicians, physician groups can create the critical mass necessary to attract managed care plan contracts and compete effectively. With broad coverage, the group can attract more managed care contracts, gain market share, and consequently gain clout. Physician groups have developed a number of network expansion strategies, including merging into larger groups; developing independent practice associations (IPAs) and physician/hospital organizations (PHOs); recruiting additional physicians, particularly primary care physicians; and affiliating with a PPMC.

Rapid Market Consolidation

Many of the players in the health care industry are consolidating rapidly in response to the continued pressure to lower health care costs. For example, HMO giant Foundation Health Systems, Inc. (formed from a merger of Health Systems International and Foundation Health Corporation), now covers over five million lives and is poised for further growth. Hospital monolith Columbia/HCA, which now owns 347 hospitals, 125 outpatient surgery centers, and 200 home health agencies, plans to develop physician networks and recently acquired a large pharmaceutical management company.

The PPMC industry is also consolidating. For example, in 1996, MedPartners purchased CareMark (September 1996), Mullikin Medical Enterprises (November 1996), and Pacific Physician Services, Inc. (February 1996), and became the largest PPMC, holding contracts with 8,875 physicians and providing prepaid care to 1.6 million people. The other PPMC powerhouse, PhyCor, has contracts with 3,240 physicians and manages IPAs representing over 9,300 physicians.

The consolidation of other players in the market can put physicians at a competitive disadvantage. Although physicians historically have preferred to practice independently, they have already begun to consolidate in response to these pressures. However, in 1995, 65.2% of nonfederal physicians still practiced in groups of less than three.

As managed care penetration increases in some markets, observers believe that physicians will consolidate to maintain leverage. Although in 1995 groups with more than 25 physicians represented only 5% of the physician groups, by the year 2000 these groups are expected to make up as much as 40% of all physician groups.

Lack of Business Experience

Many physicians are deeply troubled that the current environment seems to demand that they have the skills of an MBA; after all, they spent years in rigorous training to practice medicine, not run a business. However, because the health care system is increasingly dominated by entities that are run like businesses and routinely take steps to respond to their market, physicians must become more business savvy. They need not necessarily take time from practice, but at minimum they should obtain sound business advice from qualified professionals. Particularly in markets where capitated reimbursement becomes the norm, traditional business concepts are critical to survival.

For example, although historically physicians have distributed net income from their practice to themselves, in the current environment, most financial experts recommend that physicians retain earnings in the clinic to create an equity cushion and to provide capital for, among other things, information systems and practice expansion.

The Administrative Challenges of Capitation

Capitation is a system of payment whereby a physician or physician group agrees to provide a comprehensive set of services on a prepaid, per-member per-month basis. In essence, the physicians take on insurance risk. This can pose an enormous challenge to even the most effective clinic administrators. Although the traditional tasks of billing, collection, and controlling overhead remain critical, capitation requires additional skills and experience, most notably in managed care contract negotiation and actuarial analysis.

Developing a managed care infrastructure also involves the investment in information technology and financial systems that allow a physician group to properly price its risk. For example, accepting insurance risk requires a practice to calculate down to the penny the cost of every CPT code it bills, to establish systems that will alert the practice when costs are exceeding income, and to establish reserves for future adverse developments.

Physicians' Responses to the Changing Health Care Marketplace

A variety of options are available to physicians in the changing marketplace. Before we take an in-depth look at PPMCs, we provide a brief overview of two basic strategies for achieving the goal of building a sustainable enterprise that can profitably accept capitation and other managed care payment arrangements: expanding independently and selling to a strategic partner.

Strategic Option 1: Expand Independently

Staying independent is a viable option for some physician groups, particularly those that are well capitalized and have strong leadership. Physicians typically can access capital from one or a combination of four sources. First, they can retain earnings in the practice. This means reducing physician compensation in order to build equity reserves to reinvest in the practice. Second, they can raise additional capital among themselves, typically through private stock offerings. Third, physician groups can raise capital through traditional commercial bank debt. The latter often requires the physicians to personally guarantee the bank debt and to commit a portion of their future physician compensation toward servicing the principal and interest of that debt. Finally, if the need for capital is great enough and a sufficient business plan exists, physician groups may seek capital from an independent third party, such as a venture capitalist or strategic investor. In exchange, the physicians typically offer the funding source some form of ownership in the physician enterprise.

Exhibit 1.1 poses some questions for consideration that might help you to determine if independent expansion is the best strategic option for your group practice.

Exhibit 1.1: Is Your Clinic a Candidate for Independent Expansion?

	Yes	No	Maybe
Does the clinic have strong physician and management leadership?	☐	☐	☐
Does the clinic have a sound, well-developed, long-term business plan endorsed by physicians?	☐	☐	☐
Can clinic leadership make decisions quickly?	☐	☐	☐
Do physicians have a strong desire to maintain autonomy?	☐	☐	☐
Does the clinic have access to internally or externally generated capital?	☐	☐	☐
Is the clinic focused on "organizational wealth" instead of "personal wealth"?	☐	☐	☐
Does the clinic have a sophisticated infrastructure to support capitated contracts?	☐	☐	☐

As with most endeavors, there are both advantages and challenges associated with independent expansion. We list some of the more obvious below.

Advantages to Independent Expansion

- Ownership control is maintained.

- Operational autonomy and management consistency are ensured.

- Maximum future strategic flexibility is provided.

Challenges to Independent Expansion

- Significant capital investment in management, infrastructure, and reserves is required.

- Obtaining capital from commercial lenders, strategic partners, or venture capitalists may reduce physician compensation and dilute governance and ownership.

The following case study provides an actual example of a group practice that opted to expand its clinic independently.

Case Study: Austin Regional Clinic

The Austin Regional Clinic (ARC), a 108-physician clinic in Austin, Texas, is an example of a group that has succeeded by expanding independently. The clinic, which has 77 primary care physicians and 12 satellite locations, currently serves approximately 125,000 individual patients annually, of whom 65,000 are enrolled in HMOs.

ARC wanted to position itself as an integrated primary care–based multispecialty physician group capable of providing care under capitated arrangements in Austin, a mature managed care market with 30% HMO penetration and 35% PPO penetration. To achieve its goal, ARC successfully implemented the management and information systems needed to accept such capitated contracts. As competition in the market increased, ARC realized it needed to further develop its information systems capacity and expand its network coverage in the Austin market. The clinic looked to raise capital from a strategic partner while retaining its independence.

After exploring a number of options, including PPMC affiliation, in September 1995 ARC announced that it had secured a line of credit for an undisclosed amount from Seton Hospital to fund the clinic's strategic initiatives. ARC was able to secure capital financing from this local hospital with commercially competitive financing terms and without giving up ownership interest in the clinic or entering into any long-term contractual alliances with the hospital.

The success of this transaction is tied to ARC's ability to properly integrate its physicians into a system that was developed specifically for managed care risk contracting. ARC did everything right: it retained earnings, hired a chief operating officer (COO) with an MBA from the University of Chicago, recruited a health care industry chief financial officer (CFO), and hired an information systems consultant as its chief information officer (CIO). In addition, ARC has a full-time physician chief executive officer (CEO) who is well regarded by all health care executives in the Austin market. Today, ARC commands significant power in its market while maintaining complete independence.

Strategic Option 2: Sell to a Strategic Partner

This option involves selling the group practice to a third party, including other group practices, hospitals, health plans, and PPMCs. Exhibit 1.2 poses questions for consideration that might help you to determine if selling to a strategic partner is the best option for your group practice.

Exhibit 1.2: Is Your Clinic a Candidate for Sale to a Strategic Partner?

	Yes	No	Maybe
Are the clinic's management resources and infrastructure sufficient to profitably take capitation?	☐	☐	☐
Is the clinic capable of changing its governance structure to effectively react to changing business conditions?	☐	☐	☐
Are physician shareholders looking for liquidity?	☐	☐	☐
Is the physician panel too small or too specialist dominated to attract HMO contracts?	☐	☐	☐
Does the clinic lack access to the capital needed to position itself for managed care?	☐	☐	☐

As with the option of expanding independently, selling to a strategic partner also presents various advantages and challenges. The most obvious are outlined below.

Advantages of Selling to a Strategic Partner

- The long-term competitive position of the clinic as part of a larger, more diverse organization is enhanced.

- Clinic shareholders may convert equity value in the clinic into liquid assets such as cash or publicly traded common stock.

- The clinic gains access to the buyer's infrastructure, capital, information systems, and management resources.

Challenges of Selling to a Strategic Partner

- Physician owners relinquish control of the clinic; physician input into governance will be diluted.

- Physician compensation will initially be reduced by the management fee.

- Clinical autonomy may be diminished.

- Long-term viability of the strategic partner may be uncertain. This is especially applicable to PPMCs because of the infancy of the PPMC industry.

PPMCs as Strategic Partners

PPMCs have attracted a great deal of attention from a variety of sources. Physicians who want to relieve themselves of the burden of administration and to capitalize on the value of their existing practice are curious about opportunities to affiliate with PPMCs. Other physicians fear that the rapid growth of PPMCs may ultimately undercut physician autonomy. Wall Street has also shown intense interest in the growth prospects of PPMCs, with analysts predicting that the strong PPMCs can realize significant stock price appreciation over the next two to three years.

No comprehensive surveys of physician experience with PPMCs exist yet. Anecdotally, some physicians report high levels of satisfaction with PPMCs, while others, who may have been initially enthusiastic, have voiced reservations. Also, some PPMCs have faltered because they could not maintain their financial or market strength, strategic focus, or investor confidence. This affects affiliated physicians in a number of ways, which will be explored in chapter 3.

As you consider whether a PPMC is the best strategic partner for you, keep the following caveats in mind.

Exercise Caution

A decision to affiliate with a PPMC should be carefully thought out and well reasoned. Refrain from turning to PPMCs when you are angry, frustrated, or desperate with your existing situation because you will be more likely to agree to conditions that will be unpalatable in the future, such as noncompete clauses, limits on clinical decision making, and unfavorable practice valuations.

Establish Your Own Strategic Direction

Determine your long-term goals and objectives before you approach a PPMC. Ask yourself hard questions. What are your strengths? What do you want your practice to look like in five years? What are your weaknesses, and how would a PPMC address these weaknesses?

Identify Your Paramount Issues

Identify the issues that are nonnegotiable. Typical issues include the desire to maintain clinical autonomy, maintenance of certain levels of clinical and administrative support, stability of the PPMC, security of the consideration paid for your practice, and the ability to withdraw from the arrangement.

Develop Contingency Plans

Consider the extent to which you would be comfortable should your strategic partner change its corporate focus, merge with another PPMC, and/or sell the practice to another PPMC. Then plan for those possibilities.

Determine the Trust Level

Not every concern or contingency can be dealt with in a written legal document. Much of the success of a PPMC arrangement will depend on the degree of trust that can be established at the outset between you and the PPMC.

Conduct Your Own Due Diligence

Devote as much effort to assessing the potential PPMC partner as it will expend assessing your practice. Be sure to look at the following:

Corporate Philosophy To what extent is the PPMC's mission attuned to physician needs? Are physicians involved in decision making and to what degree?

Strategic Plan What business is the PPMC really in, and what do they expect to be involved in five years from now?

Background of the Company Principals What is the experience of the company's top executives? What has been their business success? What is their experience in running a PPMC?

Capitalization To what extent is the PPMC dependent on the stock market for its success? Does it have the ability to ride out market downturns or to finance a transition to new ventures and still continue to honor the capital obligations it proposes to make in your clinic?

Track Record with Physicians How long have the PPMC's arrangements with physicians been in place? How satisfied are participating physicians?

Market Flexibility How willing is the PPMC to tailor its approach to fit your specific practice needs? How flexible is its approach to meeting specific market demands? How willing is the PPMC to work with physicians in concert with other health care organizations, such as local hospitals?

Profitability Has the PPMC been profitable in its core services? Has it enhanced profitability of its physician practices? What are stock analysts' expectations for the PPMC's future profitability?

Answering these questions is an important start to evaluating affiliation with a PPMC. Physicians also need to assess the unique circumstances that characterize their markets and practices. The next chapter will provide a more detailed and exhaustive set of checklists to help in this evaluation.

2 The Pros and Cons of Physician Practice Management Company Affiliation

Physician groups affiliate with PPMCs for a number of reasons:

- They are aware of the push for cost containment in the health care industry.

- They want their practices to run more smoothly (which requires information systems and nonmedical personnel).

- They want to spend more time practicing medicine and less time on management tasks.

- They seek additional—and more favorable—managed care contracts.

- They need information systems to help them keep track of their performance and report the patient information and utilization rates required under managed care contracts.

In addition, many physicians practicing in a managed care environment want to gain a strategic advantage by managing risk. However, managing risk requires economies of scale, sophisticated information systems, case management expertise, and financial reserves. To accomplish this goal, many physicians need a strategic partner. One option is selling to or contracting with a PPMC.

PPMCs can help physicians accomplish these goals. However, because PPMCs are still a relatively new phenomenon, their long-term effectiveness is difficult to predict. This chapter explores both the advantages and disadvantages of affiliation with a PPMC, summarized in the following list.

Advantages

- Access to capital

- Management infrastructure and experience

- Expansion of existing business

- Overhead economies

- Relationships with managed care companies

- Operational knowledge from multiple geographic regions

- Possible physician-driven culture of PPMCs

- Opportunity for equity ownership in a larger company

Disadvantages

- For-profit character of PPMCs

- Volatile financial market conditions

- Uncertain ability to add value to physician practices

- Loss of independence

Advantages of PPMC Affiliation

Access to Capital

Physician groups seek capital for a number of reasons, including investing in managed care information systems, recruiting or acquiring additional primary care physicians, and hiring more experienced clinic administrators. Unlike most physician groups, PPMCs can access capital by selling stock in the public market or through funding from venture capital firms. Since 1993, publicly traded PPMCs have raised over $5 billion in the public markets (see Exhibit 2.1). PPMCs use this capital to fund their acquisitions and to invest in infrastructure. Venture capitalist interest in health care–related investment is on the increase, with venture capital firms investing over $1.6 billion in health care–related interests in 1996.

PPMCs usually dedicate capital each year for use by affiliated physician groups to fund their growth and development. For example, when PhyCor acquired the Arnett Clinic in August 1995, it agreed to provide the clinic with expansion capital equal to 30% of PhyCor's operating cash flow, based on PhyCor's 1995 results, or roughly $18 million, without charge.

Management Infrastructure and Experience

Some physician groups are attracted to PPMCs because they offer relief from the administrative and operational burdens of managed care. Proponents of PPMCs argue that by relieving this burden, PPMCs allow physicians to refocus

---

Exhibit 2.1: Increasing Capital Investment

---

a. Total Capital Raised by Public PPM Companies

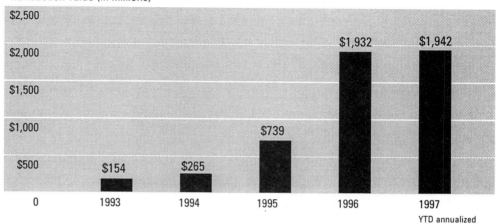

b. Health Care Venture Capital Activity

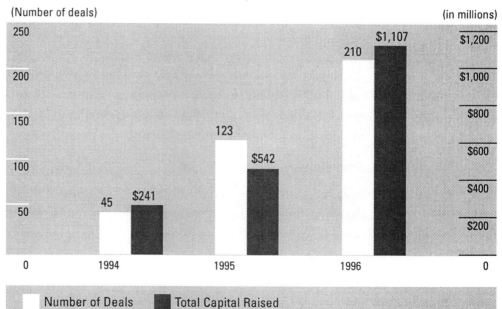

Sources: a. Townsend Frew & Co. and Securities Data Company for 1993–1997 data. 1997 data includes companies that have filed for offerings that are expected to be completed in 1997.
b. Venture One Corp. and Coopers & Lybrand.

on their primary objective, practicing medicine. PPMCs provide a range of administrative services to physician group practices. In most cases, the PPMC employs all nonprovider personnel and implements systems to handle billing, claims administration, and additional administration associated with managed care. PPMCs can also provide clinical managed care expertise by helping the physician group to develop the necessary information systems to benchmark practice patterns and underwrite profitable contracts. Many PPMCs seek to implement these high-technology systems in all of their affiliated clinics, attempting to also take advantage of preferred vendor relationships with various information systems providers.

PPMCs also help clinics develop quality assurance and utilization review protocols to profitably handle managed care. By affiliating with a PPMC, physicians also benefit from the PPMC's knowledge and experience in negotiating with managed care plans and gain negotiating leverage from being part of a larger organization.

Physicians can access similar administrative and information system assistance through other methods, primarily from an internally developed management services organization (MSO) or through outsourcing to a third-party company that provides such services. In either case, the MSO becomes largely responsible for the day-to-day operations of the clinic and the development of information systems and managed care contracting strategies. Under any of the three methods mentioned above, there is a capital outlay either in the form of management fees (paid by the physician group to PPMCs or the third-party MSOs) or in increased overhead investment in a homegrown MSO.

Expansion of Existing Business

In some markets, physician groups can better position themselves to gain control of their market by expanding the size and scope of the physician network and related services. Most PPMCs share a commitment to expanding their affiliated clinics because this serves to strengthen and increase the value of their investment as well as that of the affiliated physicians. For example, most PPMCs employ a strategy of adding new physicians (generally primary care) to an affiliated clinic to better position the clinic for larger scale managed care contracts. The PPMC will provide financial and strategic assistance in acquiring or recruiting physicians.

As a clinic considers and forms partner relationships, the clinic culture will inevitably change, and depending on the negotiated governance structure, the individual physician's voice may be diluted. Therefore, physician groups considering affiliation with a PPMC need to determine precisely how recruitment decisions will be made. Although growth in the network coverage of the clinic makes the group more attractive to HMOs, if physicians with no historical practice are recruited, financial guarantees often must be made, which can cut into physician compensation.

PPMCs also assist their affiliated clinics with the development of ancillary services such as laboratory, diagnostic, and pharmacy. Developing these services can increase patient satisfaction and *generate additional revenue* for the clinic and its physicians. However, these services must be carefully tailored to avoid violating federal anti-fraud and abuse laws.

As potential future stockholders in a publicly traded PPMC, physicians have a strong interest in seeing that the PPMC expands locally and nationally because strategic growth and resulting earnings per share increases are generally rewarded with higher stock prices. Therefore, physicians considering affiliation with a PPMC must be comfortable with the PPMC's long-term strategy. From a financial standpoint, an overextended PPMC that pays high purchase prices for practices and adds little operational value could spell trouble, or even disaster, for the PPMC and its shareholders in the future.

Overhead Economies

Some groups align with a PPMC because they believe they can leverage the PPMC's purchasing relationships and obtain better pricing for goods and services. Because of their size and scope, many PPMCs have national purchasing agreements at discounted rates for products such as medical equipment and supplies, pharmaceuticals, professional liability insurance, and office supplies. PPMCs also generate overhead savings by centralizing administrative functions such as billing and collections, scheduling, and systems management.

Relationships with Managed Care Companies

Many experts believe that physicians will benefit from consolidation by getting greater negotiating clout with health plans. Although physicians may not require strategic partners to take advantage of this shift, they will need strong management with experience in negotiating and administering managed care contracts. For physician groups that lack this internally, PPMCs may be an appealing option.

Proponents of PPMCs believe they can provide greater negotiating clout with managed care organizations.

- Most PPMCs aggressively seek managed care contracts for their physician groups, with an objective of stabilizing, if not enhancing, patient flow to the clinics.

- Most PPMCs work with a wide range of managed care organizations in a variety of markets, and this experience can benefit affiliated physicians.

- PPMCs with a statewide network can secure managed care contracts for all their affiliated groups in a region, where the clinics alone would not have such leverage.

- PPMCs can negotiate more attractive contract terms, including better premium rates.

- PPMCs may also negotiate to handle the utilization review (UR) and quality assurance (QA) for the managed care plan.

Operational Knowledge from Multiple Geographic Regions

Most PPMCs have operations in more than one market, providing physician groups access to benchmarking data, especially in the area of physician practice patterns. Some PPMCs have educational programs that highlight the most successful initiatives undertaken by affiliated clinics in the areas of medical management and transitioning to managed care.

While benchmarking against regional and national standards is helpful, the PPMC must also understand the local market. Because the dynamics of health care delivery vary dramatically by market, physicians should be leery of any partner that does not appear in tune with their market. What works in Chicago will not necessarily work in rural Texas.

Physician-Driven Culture of PPMCs

When choosing a PPMC, many physicians are more comfortable affiliating with a physician-led PPMC. Around 60% of the publicly traded PPMCs can claim that they are physician led because they have a physician CEO or chairman of the board. However, physicians must look deeper to determine whether the PPMC is, in fact, physician friendly. Before affiliating with a PPMC, a physician must carefully review the PPMC governance structure to ensure that physicians have significant input into policies affecting medical decision making, and where appropriate, corporate policy. The physician should talk to colleagues who are affiliated with the PPMC to ensure the PPMC supports independent clinical decision making. The physician should also talk to colleagues who considered, but did not choose, affiliation with the PPMC. A true physician-friendly culture can ease the transition of joining a PPMC.

Opportunity for Equity Ownership in a Larger Company

From a shareholder position, becoming part of a larger company provides the physician with the opportunity to diversify his or her risk away from a single practice/single market setting. Alignment with a PPMC allows a physician's position to change from ownership in a smaller, local business to equity ownership in a larger national company with access to capital through public and private markets. Some PPMCs have enjoyed high growth rates. This growth benefits affiliated physician shareholders who see increases in the stock prices of the equity securities they received in consideration for their affiliation. Proponents of PPMCs claim that having an equity ownership stake also serves to align the incentives of both the physician group and the management company since the entire entity benefits from profitable performance. However, physicians need to remember that the value of their investment is dependent on the performance of the stock. If the stock does not perform well, their investment will decline, possibly below levels at which the stock was received.

Disadvantages of PPMC Affiliation

While PPMCs appear to offer many attractive options for a physician group, it is necessary to understand some of the areas in which newly acquired physicians have found difficulties.

For-Profit Character of PPMCs

There is an ongoing debate over medicine as a for-profit versus not-for-profit industry. Opponents of for-profit health care companies argue that the primary goal of a for-profit corporation—to generate earnings and increase the value of the company—is in direct conflict with the physician's primary responsibility to serve as the patient's advocate. They believe that the for-profit structure provides subtle incentives to limit patient care and compromises the physician's role in patient care. They are also highly critical of the high salaries paid to many for-profit health care company executives.

Proponents of for-profit health care companies argue that there is no evidence that for-profit companies provide a lesser quality of care than not-for-profit companies and that, in fact, for-profits are run more efficiently. No definitive reports currently exist on whether there are differences between the quality of care provided by for-profit and not-for-profit companies, and the debate promises to continue. Physicians considering affiliation with a publicly traded

PPMC must determine for themselves whether they are comfortable with the for-profit culture.

Volatile Financial Market Conditions

Physicians also need to recognize that the financial markets for PPMCs are highly volatile and that sudden changes in stock price value due to fluctuations in investor sentiment and PPMC earnings are not uncommon. These fluctuations occur for several reasons.

Inability to Maintain Earnings Momentum The PPMC market has been characterized by high earnings growth rates (as high as 35% per annum). In large part, PPMCs support their growth rates through new physician practice acquisitions, which increases the risk that earnings expectations will not be met. The largest price reactions have occurred when a company has not met analysts' earnings-per-share expectations. For example, on the day that Physician Reliance Network, Inc., and MedCath Inc.—two publicly traded, single-specialty PPMCs—announced lower than expected earnings results for the third quarter of 1996, they experienced 49% and 26% declines, respectively, in their stock prices.

Rising Practice Valuations Some observers believe that the competition for the more attractive physician groups has caused overall acquisition prices to rise to levels that may jeopardize the ability of the PPMC to immediately make new acquisitions add to their earnings per share. There is pressure on a PPMC to rapidly integrate new physician practices in order that synergies obtained from integration can make the new acquisition additive to earnings per share.

Competition for Control The intense competition between providers and health plans for control of the quickly evolving health care delivery system also contributes to market volatility. Under the assumption that health care expenditures will remain flat in the future, there is a "zero sum" game at work. Said another way, one competitor's gains will almost always result in another's losses.

These market dynamics make prediction of the future earnings of PPMCs increasingly difficult. Continued volatility and earnings growth that is below expectations may dampen investors' interest in the PPMC sector and, in turn, may limit access to the capital so critical to future growth.

Uncertain Ability to Add Value to Physician Practices

While the ability of PPMCs to consolidate physician groups is clear, it is unclear whether PPMCs can run their affiliated groups more efficiently and productively than prior to acquisition over the long term. PPMCs are a new phenomenon: the oldest PPMCs are less than five years old, and most PPMCs are less than two years old. Consequently, data are insufficient to measure the efficiency of the operating structures that PPMCs bring to physician groups. Suffice it to say, however, that a PPMC with an inappropriate or inefficient operating structure will be unsustainable over the long term in the increasingly competitive health care market.

Loss of Independence

Physicians choosing PPMCs as partners face several major transitions upon the close of the acquisition transaction. First, physicians will have to transition from an independent setting, in which their income was based on the number of procedures they performed, to a PPMC arrangement where they receive a salary, a percentage of which may be based on performance measures. Second, physicians will share governance of their practice in a 50-50 arrangement with the PPMC. The organization will now make the clinic's business decisions within the context of financial and operating budgets as well as minimum return on invested capital. Physicians and the PPMC will share the decisions about which managed care organizations to pursue. Third, the decision to add or remove physicians from the clinic will be much less a matter of collegiality and personal economics as a matter of what best positions the clinic to compete for large-scale managed care contracts. Finally, physicians who choose to affiliate with a PPMC must be willing to participate in PPMC-directed quality management and utilization review initiatives and to participate in the training and implementation of procedural protocols.

Physicians, in general, will feel the pressure of meeting quarter-to-quarter earnings goals that results from the public status of the PPMC (although some PPMCs are privately held entities).

In the next chapter we take a closer look at the organizational structure and various models of PPMCs. We also examine some of the acquisition, operating, and growth trends in the industry.

3 Organizational Structure of Physician Practice Management Companies

PPMCs are classified by their affiliation design and by their physician mix (see Exhibit 3.1). Affiliation design describes the method a PPMC uses to associate with physicians. Physician mix refers to the types of physicians in which the PPMC chooses to affiliate. For example, PhyCor, Inc., is a PPMC that uses the equity model affiliation design as its primary means of partnering with multispecialty physician groups. This chapter provides an overview of these structures.

Exhibit 3.1: PPMC Organizational Designs

By Affiliation Design

- Equity Model

- Management Company Model

- Physician Contractor Model

By Physician Mix

- Primary Care/Multispecialty

- Single Specialty

Affiliation Design

Equity Model

The equity model takes its name from the series of financial transactions that result in a PPMC offering a purchase price to the physician shareholders of a clinic in return for an equity stake by the PPMC in the ongoing revenue and cash flows of the clinic. The most common form of equity model PPMC involves two major events:

- The PPMC purchases the clinic's tangible assets, excluding real estate.

- A long-term (generally 25 to 40 years) management services agreement between the PPMC and the clinic is executed.

While there are structuring exceptions, which are largely driven by tax planning, in the equity model typically a local subsidiary corporation of the PPMC is established. This corporation purchases the assets of the clinic and also assumes all nonphysician personnel into its payroll.

Simultaneously, the management services agreement is executed between the PPMC and the clinic, which generally retains its identity as a professional association (P.A.) or professional corporation (P.C.). The physicians remain employees of the P.A. and sign employment agreements (generally three to five years) with noncompete provisions. In addition, the management agreement calls for a certain percentage of the local subsidiary's income after operating expenses, but before physician compensation, to be paid to the PPMC as the "management fee."

The PPMC uses the anticipated pro forma stream of earnings that is the management fee to determine the value it is willing to pay to purchase the clinic enterprise, which includes value of the assets. As a general rule, PPMCs seek to purchase clinics at a multiple of five to eight times pro forma first-year management fees.

Consideration for such transactions generally comes as a mix. Few transactions are 100% cash or 100% stock in the PPMC. Most are a mix of cash, the assumption of selected liabilities, notes from the PPMC, and stock in the PPMC.

Once the clinic is acquired, the PPMC assumes the clinic's administrative functions, allowing the physicians to concentrate on the practice of medicine. Services provided by PPMCs for the clinic can include equipment and facility maintenance, management information systems, billing and collections, strategic planning, budgeting, and the development of managed care relationships. Because the equity model generally aligns the incentives of the PPMC and the physician, proponents believe that it tends to maximize the clinic's productivity, efficiency, and marketability.

Policy Board Both the physicians and the PPMC share governance on a joint policy board, which presides over the business and strategic planning issues of the clinic. When deciding whether to affiliate with a PPMC, physicians should assess carefully the makeup and duties of the governance board to ensure that they are comfortable with the ability of this body to appropriately influence the ongoing operations of the clinic. In general, the makeup of the governance board is three members from the PPMC (one of whom can be the clinic's current administrator) and three physician members from the clinic (typically from different departments). Duties of the policy board can include hiring physicians and administrators, setting patient fee schedules, determining capital improvements and expansion, and evaluating provider and payer relationships.

Potential for Future Value Physician shareholders can benefit in two ways from increased future value as a result of an equity affiliation. The first opportunity comes from an upside appreciation in the value of any stock held in the PPMC that physician shareholders might have taken as part of the purchase price consideration. The second opportunity for increased value is realized if the PPMC increases revenues and utilizes expense more efficiently than the clinic would have been able to achieve on its own. Whether value comes from stock price appreciation or the specific operations of the clinic, physicians will benefit.

Potential Risk In an effort to balance this discussion, we must note that there is also downside potential in the general risk one takes in owning equity. If the stock of the PPMC slides due to reasons beyond the control of the clinic, the physicians will have lost value from where they started at the close of the affiliation transaction. In the same vein, if the PPMC is unable to add operational value to the clinic beyond what the physicians could have achieved on their own, then 40 years of a management fee in comparison to the consideration received for purchase may be economically adverse to the physicians.

Management Company Model

In the management company model, physicians maintain their independent practices, and the PPMC does not acquire the clinic or its assets or seek to enter into a long-term agreement. Instead the PPMC affiliates through a shorter term management contract. Management company PPMCs are attractive to clinics whose highest perceived need is for additional revenue in the form of profitable managed care contracts.

Management company model PPMCs fall into two types, which we discuss below: those that provide network management (IPA management companies) and those that provide practice management expertise. IPA management companies, the newest form of management company, direct the IPA's contracts with managed care payers, while practice management companies also direct the activities at the heart of the day-to-day practice, such as scheduling, billing, and collections.

IPA Management Companies As a response to managed care, many physicians have affiliated with one or more independent practice associations (IPAs). An IPA allows a physician to maintain an independent practice while gaining leverage with managed care plans by affiliating with other physicians to negotiate managed care contracts. The goal of IPAs is to provide physicians with a common infrastructure to perform profitably in a managed care environment, which is especially important when such contracts' reimbursement patterns are shifting from discounted fee-for-service to capitation. Although some observers predicted that IPAs would not survive because they cannot compete with tightly integrated physician group models, they continue to flourish in many parts of the country (see Exhibit 3.2).

Exhibit 3.2: Percentage of Physicians Affiliated with IPAs, 1991–1995

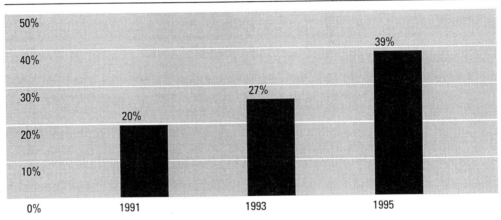

Source: Modern Physician, October 1996.

In its most general form, the relationship between the IPA and the management company is that of client/vendor. The IPA (the client) pays a fee, typically a percentage of contract revenue that flows through the IPA, to the management company (the vendor) for services. As a larger entity with larger purchasing power, the IPA management company is able to achieve economies of scale that keep costs lower than any single-proprietor operation could possibly achieve.

The IPA management company affiliates with an individual IPA through a short-term management contract. In addition to providing administrative functions, the PPMC's role is to help the IPA attract and negotiate beneficial HMO contracts. By managing a broad network of IPAs, the PPMC can often leverage its various geographical affiliations into a network that attracts managed care contracts on a regional basis.

Practice Managment Expertise Providers While network management companies, for the most part, focus on revenue enhancement, practice management companies focus on clinic expense savings. Practice management companies will provide payroll, billing and collections, human resources, and other services to physician groups for a set fee (usually on a percentage basis). By performing these services more efficiently than physicians are able to, practice management groups are able to save physician clinics money. To date, this has largely been a cottage industry with many small players.

Physician Contractor Model

Physician contractor PPMCs provide physician services primarily to hospitals. The PPMC contracts with physicians, generally on an independent contractor basis, to provide the desired services to a hospital. The PPMC's contracts with the hospital typically have terms of three years but can be terminated by either party with 90 days written notice. Independent contractor physicians generally receive a base salary plus a productivity bonus based on Relative Value Units (RVUs). This model is distinct from the previous two models in that the primary goal is to ease the hospital's burden by administering and operating certain departments. Hospital emergency departments most commonly outsource services to PPMCs and other entities, but increasingly hospitals out-source other practice areas, such as radiology, anesthesiology, and neonatology.

Examples of publicly traded PPMCs using the physician contractor model include Pediatrix Medical Group; EmCare, Inc.; Coastal Physician Group, Inc.; and InPhyNet Medical Management, Inc., which is in the process of being acquired by MedPartners.

Exhibit 3.3 provides some suggestions on how one or another model of PPMC might fit your practice.

Exhibit 3.3: Which Type of PPMC Fits Your Practice?

If you are . . .	You might consider . . .
An emergency room physician who values your independence . . .	Becoming an independent contractor to a physician contractor model PPMC
A larger group that needs expertise, wants to get the value for its equity, is not terribly concerned about remaining independent, and wants a partner . . .	Affiliating with an equity model PPMC

| A physician group that just needs revenue and/or some help with its expense management because there are inefficiencies in the clinic operations . . . | Affiliating with a management company model PPMC |

Physician Mix

Primary Care/Multispecialty

Very few PPMCs acquire only primary care clinics (PCPs) because relative to multispecialty practices, this type of clinic does not generate the revenues that allow PPMCs to show quarterly growth or gain the critical mass to go public. Therefore, almost all PPMCs start out by affiliating with multispecialty groups, then moving toward a much stronger concentration of primary care physicians in the total physician mix. Because PCPs play a more prominent role in managing and directing health care expenditures under managed care, most equity model PPMCs, including MedPartners and PhyCor, believe that primary care–driven multispecialty groups are the best positioned to control the market. These PPMCs pursue this strategy for several reasons:

- Multispecialty clinics are attractive to patients because they offer a wide range of primary, specialty, and ancillary services in a single location with significant market control.

- Multispecialty clinics are favored by managed care organizations because of the large number and variety of services the clinics provide and the expectation that multispecialty clinics can control hospital utilization and total health care costs more effectively.

- Multispecialty clinics can provide an extensive range of health care services in an ambulatory setting, thereby reducing treatment costs and capitalizing on the trend of shifting patient care to alternative sites.

- Multispecialty clinics allow physicians to pool their resources to finance medical equipment, technology, and support services not typically available to physicians in smaller group settings.

On the other hand, physicians in multispecialty/primary care groups are affiliating with PPMCs for a number of reasons:

- They are aware of the push for cost containment in the health care industry and thus the need for larger critical mass and operating scales.

- They want their practices to run more efficiently (which requires information systems and nonmedical personnel).

- They want to spend more time practicing medicine and less time on management tasks.

- They seek additional—and more favorable—managed care contracts and are attracted to the leverage offered by PPMCs.

- They need information systems to help them keep track of their performance and report the patient information and utilization rates often required under managed care contracts.

- All of the above require capital that many groups are unable to access.

Single Specialty

Some PPMCs focus on acquiring practices with a single specialty, such as oncology, ophthalmology, orthopedics, or cardiology. Specialists consolidate into single-specialty groups because they believe that concentrating on a single disease category gives them significant competitive advantages, including the ability to control quality while containing costs through expertise in a specific disease category. They also believe that treating specific disease categories provides economies of scale not generally available across a broad range of disease categories. Single-specialty groups also provide capital to allow physicians to afford state-of-the-art equipment and achieve more efficient utilization of that equipment through increased volumes of patients in lower cost ambulatory settings.

Single-specialty PPMCs base their strategy on a belief that managed care organizations can ultimately recognize lower costs through contracting with organizations that possess specific carve-out expertise in high-cost areas of medicine.

Single-specialty clinics typically generate more revenue and higher operating margins than multispecialty clinics, which is attractive to a PPMC from a financial viewpoint. The average 12-month operating income margin for publicly traded single-specialty PPMCs (as of June 30, 1996) was 15.0%, compared with 4.8% for multispecialty PPMCs. An analysis of announced clinic acquisitions since 1991 shows that single-specialty clinics produced an average of $895,000 of revenue per physician while multispecialty clinics produced $543,000 per physician. PPMCs that have adopted the single-specialty clinic strategy include American Oncology Resources, Inc.; EquiMed, Inc.; and MedCath Incorporated. Single-specialty PPMCs that have recently completed public offerings include Specialty Care Network, Inc. (musculoskeletal); Specialty Corp. (ear, nose, and throat, and head and neck); and AmeriPath, Inc. (pathology).

Single-specialty groups may choose to affiliate with a PPMC for the same reasons that a multispecialty/primary care physician group would. Specialists are facing a crunch as managed care tries to limit utilization. Affiliating with a PPMC can help specialists negotiate managed care contracts and offer better assurances that they will not be cut from an HMO's network. Like physicians in multispecialty groups, specialists are encountering the increased administrative burdens of providing care in a managed care environment and uncertainty in the level of their future income. Affiliation with a PPMC can be a way to alleviate many of these concerns.

PPMC Growth and Operating Trends

Wall Street perceives the PPMC industry as an area that will offer significant earnings growth opportunities because of demonstrated high price-to-earnings (P/E) ratios. P/E ratios are calculated by dividing a company's stock price by its earnings for a given period. High P/E multiples indicate that investors believe a company's earnings can grow significantly in the future. Multispecialty/primary care PPMCs traded at an average multiple to 1997 estimated earnings of 25.2. Single-specialty PPMCs traded at an average multiple to 1997 estimated earnings of 20.1, while hospital-based PPMCs traded at an average multiple of 20.8, both for the same time period.

From January 1, 1993, through December 31, 1996, publicly traded PPMCs have experienced an average annual revenue growth rate of approximately 269%. Analysts expect this growth rate to continue over the next three to five years. Analysts also predict that PPMC earnings will increase an average of 30% over the next five years, while HMO earnings are projected to increase at only 18%, hospital earnings at 17%, and pharmaceutical company earnings at 12%.

Within the PPMC market performance varies. The single-specialty PPMCs experienced the most rapid annual revenue growth from January 1, 1993, to December 31, 1996, with a revenue increase of nearly 400%. The single-specialty PPMCs also experienced the highest operating income margins over the last 12 months, with an average 15.0% margin. However, multispecialty/primary care PPMCs are expected to grow an average of 35% over the next five years, outpacing the rest of the PPMCs.

When PPMCs Falter

Physicians considering affiliation with a PPMC should be cautioned that over time, the PPMC market will probably consolidate even further, and some PPMCs will fail. The same phenomenon is occurring now in the HMO industry, which expanded rapidly in the 1980s and is now going through intense consolidation. This trend is beginning to occur in the PPMC industry. Market volatility can have a profound impact on a physician who chooses to affiliate with a PPMC that either goes out of business or is merged into a second PPMC with a different management philosophy, from both a clinical and a financial standpoint.

For example, when physicians affiliate with a PPMC, some of the consideration they usually receive is in the form of stock in the PPMC. If a PPMC begins to perform poorly, the physician could see the value of his or her stock decline. Also, a faltering PPMC may be acquired by a different PPMC whose organizational philosophy, culture, and management varies considerably from the original PPMC. In the worst-case scenario, when the company goes out of business, the physicians will essentially have to start at square one in rebuilding a practice.

If the PPMC falters, it also may lose its ability to raise capital out in the public markets, which may put the breaks on strategic initiatives that are critical to maintaining a competitive position.

Case Study: Coastal Physician Group, Inc.

Coastal Physician Group, Inc., provides an example of the volatile nature of the PPMC market. Coastal historically followed the physician contractor model by contracting with hospitals to manage emergency departments. When Coastal went public in June 1991, it shifted its focus and began seeking out alternative sites, focusing more on primary care and multispecialty groups and less on emergency room. Coastal purchased a number of physician groups in the South, following a standard equity model approach.

At first, Coastal's stock did very well. Then, in late 1995, Coastal made what in retrospect was a major misstep. Coastal owned several practices in Florida whose sole contracts were with Humana, a large HMO. In 1995, Coastal purchased a Florida HMO, and Humana perceived Coastal to be its direct competitor, not its contract vendor.

Humana reacted by withdrawing enrollees and changing its contract with the physician groups in south Florida. Since approximately 90% of Coastal's south Florida business came from Humana, the changes reduced Coastal's profitability, and it lost significant money on its south Florida clinic operations. As a result, the company experienced an earnings strain and began a downward spiral of unmet earnings and declining stock values.

This chain of events proved disastrous to the physicians in the Florida clinics who had accepted Coastal stock as part of the affiliation transaction. Their stock, which had traded as high as $42, dropped to $4. Coastal, after weathering a proxy battle, now spends much of its time solving its bank problems instead of running the PPMC. The company is in the process of selling off many of its assets, while trying to develop a new core focus.

How to Evaluate a PPMC

Physicians considering affiliation with a PPMC must ensure that they affiliate with an entity that will survive and thrive in what could be a volatile PPMC market. They should spend time researching the PPMCs that want to acquire their practice. The following checklists outline various factors that should be considered in evaluating a PPMC for strategic partnership.

Operating Factors Checklist

√ The PPMC's management is experienced in practice management and is expert at dealing with managed care companies and their effects on physicians.

√ The PPMC has strong physician leadership, which inspires trust in physicians. The governance structure allows for significant physician input and for clinical autonomy.

√ The PPMC can bring valuable operational efficiencies to the acquired clinic, such as a strong information technology system that provides efficient administration and billing, tracks cost and clinical data, monitors and profiles providers, and allows for longitudinal data collection and dissemination.

√ The PPMC can secure and profitably handle managed care contracts. It can position the acquired clinics to take on managed care from an operational standpoint, including positioning the clinics to take on global capitation in the states in which that is allowed.

√ The PPMC accurately projects earnings per share. This is critical to the PPMC's success, because its stock price can decline sharply if it misses an estimate by as little as a penny. When companies report their quarterly earnings, they usually announce whether they hit their earnings estimates.

√ The PPMC's stock price does not fluctuate wildly. If it does, the physician probably does not want to be affiliated with that PPMC.

Acquisition Execution and Integration Checklist

√ The PPMC uses a sound acquisition model and a disciplined valuation approach. Successful PPMCs acquire clinics that will build and diversify their revenue base, advance their business strategy, and pay fair market value for those clinics. They are also proficient at integrating the newly acquired clinics into the company by assimilating them on the same computer systems and providing the same services to the newly acquired clinic that the existing clinics receive.

√ The PPMC involves the local physicians in clinic governance. A clinic will not succeed unless physicians have a sense of ownership and control over the direction of the clinic and their clinical decision making.

√ The PPMC has a good reputation and a consistent operating history. These will help the PPMC attract new clinics. The PPMC's ability to acquire new clinics is a leading indicator of its future growth.

Challenges Facing PPMCs

PPMCs face challenges in order to survive and thrive in the competitive marketplace. For example, when a PPMC makes acquisitions in several states, it must integrate all its physician groups with its existing operations. PPMCs must also be good managers of the physicians they acquire by giving them a voice in clinic operations and by keeping their morale high. PPMCs that are not effective managers of capitation also will be at a disadvantage. An unprofitable managed care contract can financially devastate the PPMC. Because of the many variables that lead to success in the PPMC market, physicians must carefully evaluate whether affiliation with a particular PPMC is a wise strategy.

4 PPMC Acquisitions of Physician Services

In this chapter we move beyond the basic characteristics of PPMCs to address in more depth how PPMCs acquire physician group practices. First, we address the two different types of acquisitions: pooling of interests and purchase of assets. Then we examine the common elements of an acquisition transaction. In order to make this information as understandable as possible, we will walk through a typical acquisition performed by an equity model PPMC.

We must emphasize that as far as acquisition transactions go, no two transactions are exactly alike. Each deal, depending on the players, the practice, and the particular situation, is different.

Following our discussion of PPMC acquisitions, we will briefly address current acquisition trends.

Practice Acquisition Transaction Types

A PPMC, when it acquires a physician group practice, structures the transaction as either a pooling of interests or as a purchase of assets. The type and related structure of an acquisition transaction are of great importance to the PPMC because they affect its financial and accounting statements. The type of transaction that is performed is also of significance to the medical practice being acquired because it affects the nature of the consideration that is paid to the owners of the practice.

Pooling of Interests

In a pooling-of-interests transaction, the two companies involved merge their respective assets, liabilities, and operating results without changes or adjustments. The financial statements of the companies are combined as though the companies had always been commonly owned. The acquired practice becomes a part of the acquiring PPMC, and the historical financial statements of the PPMC are then restated to reflect the results of the combined organizations after the pooling of interests.

In this type of transaction, the law and the Generally Accepted Accounting Principles (GAAP) utilized by accountants require that consideration paid to the group practice must be substantially in the form of common stock. No more than 10% of the consideration may include cash, notes, or earnouts. Earnouts are compensation paid to the physicians in the form of bonuses when certain financial goals are met. For example, the goals might involve the practice generating a certain amount of revenue or achieving certain levels of cost containment.

A transaction must meet several stringent legal and accounting requirements in order to qualify as a pooling of interests. These requirements state that:

- Each party (i.e., the PPMC and the practice) must have been independent and autonomous companies for two years prior to the deal.

- The transaction must be final within one year of the definitive agreement to pool interests.

- One hundred percent of the common stock of the group practice must be exchanged for common stock of the acquiring party.

- Once there is definitive agreement to pool interests there can be no changes in the practice ownership. In other words, an outsider anticipating a quick profit at acquisition may not buy a stake in the practice.

- There can be no intent to sell significant group practice assets after the definitive agreement is completed.

Purchase of Assets

In a purchase transaction, the PPMC is identified as the acquiring company because it is purchasing the assets or stock of the target group practice for an agreed-upon price. The purchase price, after deducting the fair market value of the liabilities, is then allocated to the acquired assets. In other words, a different percentage of the purchase price is allocated to the facilities, to the equipment, to the inventory, and to other assets. Any excess money left over after allocating the purchase price to the assets is recorded as goodwill. The PPMC must amortize, or spread out, the goodwill over the approximate remaining useful life of the acquired assets (usually 20 to 40 years). The reported financial statements of the acquiring party include the financials of the target group from the date of the acquisition but do not include prior financial statements. Unlike a pooling, purchase transactions may involve any negotiated form of consideration, including cash, stock, or bonuses.

In the PPMC industry, most acquisitions have been purchase transactions. Most of the pooling transactions involve larger transactions where the amount of the goodwill is so high that the amortized expense of the goodwill would negatively impact the future earnings of the PPMC.

Since August 1991, only 33 acquisitions, or 8% of transactions during that time period, have been accounted for as a pooling of interests. Those same 33 pooling transactions, however, represent almost $3.5 billion in transaction values, or roughly 56% of the total dollar value from all acquisitions in the PPMC industry. The average acquisition value per transaction for purchase agreements is about $16 million, while the average acquisition value per transaction accounted for as a pooling of interest totals $106 million.

Acquisition Transaction Terms

With the caveat that transaction terms will vary from one acquisition to another, every acquisition includes several key elements, which we describe below.

Asset Acquisition

First, the PPMC will acquire certain assets of the practice. In some cases the PPMC acquires all or a substantial portion of the practice's assets, while in others it may be limited to only selected assets. Most PPMCs acquire all the medical assets of the clinic, such as the medical equipment; however, other assets, such as real estate, may or may not be included. Other examples of nonmedical assets are furniture and fixtures, accounts receivable, and intangible assets like goodwill or patient records.

Assumption of Liabilities

In some cases, the PPMC will also assume all or some of the liabilities associated with the practice. Liabilities are debts due and payable, such as accounts payable, taxes, and notes payable (debt financing). If a PPMC does not assume the liabilities from the practice, the current owners are responsible for meeting all obligations. These liabilities are typically resolved using the proceeds from the sale of the practice.

Liabilities may also include judgments entered against the practice in lawsuits. In most cases, legal claims against the practice stemming from a lawsuit remain the responsibility of the current owners. An acquiring purchaser is not subject to claims made against the current ownership of the practice, and these liabilities are separated from the acquisition plan.

Management Service Agreement

Simultaneous to the completion of the acquisition, the newly affiliated physician group enters into a long-term management service agreement with the PPMC. This document governs the relationship of the physician and the PPMC for the term of the agreement, which is typically anywhere from 15 to 40 years, and establishes the fee that is to be paid to the PPMC for services provided to the practice.

Under the terms of most management service agreements, the PPMC provides the affiliated group with the equipment and facilities used in the medical practice, manages all clinic operations, provides all accounting work (including billing and collections), employs the nonphysician staff, provides access to capital, and manages the payer relationships. Typically, the PPMC also provides the group with information systems, including computer hardware and software. The PPMC may also help negotiate new payer contracts, recruit new physicians, and provide ancillary services previously performed outside the practice.

Management Fee

The size of the management fee varies among PPMCs and reflects only the services that are specifically provided for by the management service agreement. The fee is commonly established as a fixed percentage of net revenues received by the group (generally 5% to 20% of total revenues less operating expenses). As shown in Exhibit 4.1, PPMC management fees can greatly affect physician compensation and place a greater emphasis on expense control.

Effect of Management Fees on Physician Compensation Exhibit 4.1 shows how the management fee charged by the PPMC affects physician compensation.

The projected income statement shows projected income prior to affiliation with a PPMC. In Year 1, the practice is forecasted to earn $10 million in revenues. The operating expenses of the clinic, which equal $5 million (or 50% of revenue), are deducted from this amount. The remaining $5 million in net revenues available to the physicians for compensation is divided by the 20 physicians in the practice, resulting in $250,000 compensation for each physician in Year 1.

The pro forma income statement after PPMC affiliation is similar to the projected income statement, but shows the addition of a management fee paid to the PPMC. In the example, the management fee is set at 15% of revenue, which equals $750,000. This amount is deducted from the net revenues of the practice. The physicians in the practice now have only $4.25 million available for compensation, and each would receive only $213,000 in Year 1.

In order to regain pre-PPMC income levels, the group practice needs to generate significant revenue growth, expense savings, or both. The philosophy of PPMCs is that the opportunities for practice growth and expense reduction afforded by the PPMC allow physicians to "earn through" the management fee within one to three years. This philosophy assumes that no major issues arise and that the group practice has chosen a PPMC that brings with it significant opportunities. There are, of course, no guarantees.

Exhibit 4.1: Effect of Management Fees on Physician Compensation

Projected Income Statement (prior to PPMC affiliation)

(dollars in thousands)	Year 1	Year 2	Year 3	Year 4
Net revenue	$10,000	$11,000	$12,100	$13,000
Clinic overhead	5,000	5,500	6,050	6,650
Percent of revenue	50%	50%	50%	50%
Net to practice	5,000	5,500	6,050	6,650
Number of physicians	20	20	20	20
Per physician compensation	$250	$275	$303	$333

Pro Forma Income Statement (after PPMC affiliation)

(dollars in thousands)	Year 1	Year 2	Year 3	Year 4
Net revenue	$10,000	$11,000	$12,100	$13,000
Clinic overhead	5,000	5,500	6,050	6,650
Percent of revenue	50%	50%	50%	50%
Net to practice	5,000	5,500	6,050	6,650
Management fee	$750	$825	$908	$998
Percent of net to practice	15%	15%	15%	15%
Available to physicians	$4,250	$4,675	$5,142	$5,652
Number of physicians	20	20	20	20
Per physician compensation	$213	$234	$257	$283
Required additional revenue to maintain pre-PPMC income	**$1,780**	**$1,950**	**$2,140**	**$2,350**

Employment Agreement

In the equity model, physicians in affiliated groups typically sign employment agreements with the PPMC for terms of three to five years. The employment agreement provides for the affiliated physicians either a flat salary or, more commonly, a certain percentage of group revenues. Part or all of the affiliated physicians' compensation may be earnouts, which are tied to the profitability of the clinic so physicians have an incentive to control costs.

If a physician were to leave the clinic upon expiration of the employment agreement, he or she would have no further obligations under the clinic's long-term management agreement. The long-term management agreement is between the clinic and the PPMC, whereas the employment contract is between the individual physician and the physician association. This arrangement enables the PPMC to provide continuous management services even if there is physician turnover.

Along with the employment agreements, the PPMC may require physicians to sign noncompete covenants, also called restrictive covenants, which prohibit affiliated physicians from competing with any other physicians or physician groups affiliated with the PPMC in a specified geographic area for a specified time period. The covenants also prohibit physicians from disclosing certain confidential and proprietary information relating to the PPMC and its affiliated physician groups.

Consideration

The consideration, or purchase price, that is paid to the group practice in exchange for acquisition of the assets of the practice usually consists of a combination of cash, stock, liability assumption, deferred purchase price payments in the form of seller notes (contractual promissory notes for payments to be made in the future), or contingent consideration (bonus payments) that is paid when certain financial goals are met. In some cases, the common stock issued by PPMCs may include a restriction that prevents its sale for up to two years, and this affects the liquidity of the investment. Generally speaking, the consideration mix of the acquisition depends on the needs and objectives of the two parties.

In the following case study we illustrate a typical acquisition transaction using PhyCor, Inc., as an example.

Case Study: PhyCor, Inc.

PhyCor, Inc., an equity model PPMC, typically acquires group practices through a purchase of assets. PhyCor purchases the operating assets of the clinic, such as accounts receivable, inventory, and equipment. Historically, PhyCor's clinic acquisitions have all been accounted for as purchase transactions valued at five to eight times the anticipated first-year earnings of the clinic before interest has been added and taxes deducted (EBIT). (We will discuss valuation approaches later in this chapter.) The consideration offered in exchange for the assets usually consists of the following:

- 20% assumed liabilities
- 20%–25% PhyCor common stock
- 10%–20% deferred purchase price payments (sellers' notes)
- 35%–50% cash

Selected transactions include earnouts, which are contingent consideration paid to clinic shareholders as bonuses if certain financial or operating targets are achieved. Such targets may consist of minimum revenue earnings or achieving a certain mix of primary care physicians in relation to the clinic's total physician panel within a specified period of time. Other transactions include provisions for a purchase price reduction in the event that any of the clinic's physicians do not execute a noncompetition agreement by the closing date.

Simultaneous to the purchase of operating assets, PhyCor and the acquired clinic enter into a long-term (usually 40 years) service agreement. In exchange for a fee, PhyCor provides the following to each of its clinics:

- Equipment and facilities
- Management of clinic operations
- Employment of nonphysician personnel
- Continuing medical education
- Capital
- Medical and managerial information systems
- Development of managed care relationships

Service agreements can be terminated only for cause, which includes material default or bankruptcy. Some service agreements grant termination rights to physicians if more than 50% of PhyCor's shares are acquired by a third party. In addition, some practices have negotiated the first right of refusal to purchase the clinic's assets if PhyCor determines to sell such assets.

Each clinic pays an annual management fee to PhyCor based upon a percent (usually 13% to 17%) of the clinic's annual net revenue less clinic operating expenses, excluding physician compensation (also called the predistribution pool). PhyCor believes that this model aligns the physicians' incentives to both grow revenues and control costs.

Each PhyCor clinic is governed by a joint policy board that has equal (50–50) representation of PhyCor management and clinic physicians. The governing structure allows physicians to maintain visibility and continue to direct the clinic. For each clinic they acquire, PhyCor appoints an executive director who is responsible for the daily operations of the clinic and for implementing the policies of the board. Because of the 50–50 mix, voting ties on decisions are not easily broken. However, industry sources state that there are rarely stalemates in PhyCor groups, which suggests that the members of the board ultimately negotiate to resolution before they make and implement decisions. Exhibit 4.2 shows PhyCor's governance chart.

Exhibit 4.2: PhyCor Governance Chart

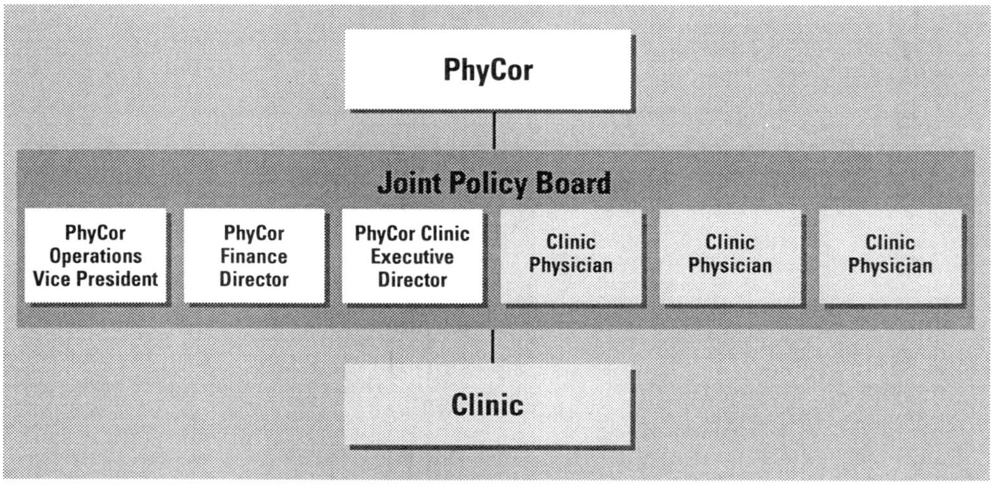

The specific duties of PhyCor's policy board include:
- Capital improvements and expansion
- Annual budgeting
- Advertising
- Patient fee schedules
- Ancillary services
- Provider/payer relationships
- Strategic planning

- Physician recruitment and hiring
- Selection of executive director
- Grievance referrals

With the success of PhyCor, other PPMCs soon followed in PhyCor's footsteps and devised their own strategies of how best to combine physician practices and corporate management. Other PPMCs, both public and private, have adopted this model for valuing and developing their own acquisition targets.

How PPMCs Value Physician Groups

If you are considering affiliation with a PPMC, you should understand how the PPMC will value your practice and determine a purchase price. While PPMCs may use any of a variety of accepted analytical methods to arrive at the value of a medical practice, generally one of two common approaches are used: the income approach or the market analysis approach.

Income Approach

The income approach to valuing a practice involves projecting the future earnings of the practice and then discounting them so that they are reflected in terms of today's dollars. The analytical method used to accomplish this, the discounted cash flow method, is not conceptually difficult to understand. However, to gain a true appreciation of all the complexities of the analysis would require a discussion beyond the scope of this book. For this reason, we offer only a summary of the method and a simplified example.

As noted, the discounted cash flow method is based on the idea that earnings generated in the future, although greater than present earnings, will have a lower value than that same amount of money today. The first step in performing a discounted cash flow analysis is to reasonably project the earnings for the practice into the future. For these purposes we will project for six years. These earnings include all fee-for-service, capitated, and shared-risk revenues.

	Year 1	Year 2	Year 3	Year 4	Year 5
Gross income	$253,000	$260,590	$268,408	$276,460	$284,754

Next, deduct the operating expenses of the practice. These operating expenses include all physician and nonphysician compensation, supplies, rent, insurance, purchased services, and other administrative expenses. The amount of money remaining is the net revenue or operating income of the practice.

	Year 1	Year 2	Year 3	Year 4	Year 5
Gross income	$253,000	$260,590	$268,408	$276,460	$284,754
Operating expense	$252,798	$255,378	$257,671	$259,872	$261,973
Operating income	$200	$5,212	$10,736	$16,588	$22,780

Because interest expense is not considered a part of the discounted cash flow calculation, we add it back into operating income total. Taxes and capital expenditures are considered in the calculation, so we deduct them from any operating income. The resulting sum, called free cash flow, serves as the basis for the present value calculation.

	Year 1	Year 2	Year 3	Year 4	Year 5
Operating income	$202	$5,212	$10,736	$16,588	$22,780
Interest (+)	$5,000	$5,000	$5,000	$5,000	$5,000
Taxes (−)	$1,977	$3,880	$5,980	$8,203	$10,557
Capital (−)	$25,000	0	0	0	0
Free cash flow	−$21,775	$6,331	$9,757	$13,384	$17,224

The discount or present value rate that is applied to the free cash flows to arrive at discounted free cash flows is a constant value that we can obtain by using a present value table (found in most financial publications) or by performing a present value calculation on a financial calculator. The discount rate is derived by two key factors: the desired return on investment (ROI) percentage and the projection period number. A common ROI percentage is 16%.

	Year 1	Year 2	Year 3	Year 4	Year 5
Free cash flows	−$21,775	$6,331	$9,757	$13,384	$17,224
Discount rate (.16)	0.8621	0.7432	0.6407	0.5523	0.4761
Present value of free cash flows	−$18,772	$4,705	$6,251	$7,392	$8,200

To complete the valuation analysis and arrive at the value of the practice, we must determine the terminal value of the practice. The terminal value of the practice, the expected worth of the practice at the end of the projection range (Year 6), is calculated by dividing the free cash flow in Year 6 by the return on investment percentage (16%):

Terminal value = $17,224 / .16 = $107,650

We then multiply the terminal value by the discount rate for Year 6 (0.4761) to arrive at the present value of the terminal value, which in our example is $51,252.

The final step in the valuation process is to add the present value of the terminal value to the sum of all the discounted free cash flows across the projection range. This results in the total value of the practice according to this valuation method.

Present value of terminal value	$51,252
Total of discounted free cash flows	$7,777
Total practice value	$59,029

Market Analysis Approach

A discounted cash flow analysis is not the only means by which a PPMC will value a potential acquisition target. PPMCs also look at market factors to determine acquisition values and may analyze acquisitions of similar targets in comparable markets made by other companies. This type of information gives a PPMC a good idea of what values other PPMCs or the market as a whole is placing on selected acquisition targets. The PPMCs generally evaluate annual total revenue, EBIT, or per physician multiples of purchase price to determine comparable acquisition values.

In addition, certain transactions may provide significant synergy or have strategic importance to PPMCs. This may increase the overall attractiveness and therefore increase the overall value of the target. While a discounted cash flow analysis is a more sophisticated way to value an acquisition, in many cases the PPMC simply pays what the market demands, whether it is at a premium or discount to the discounted cash flow valuation.

The valuation of medical practices is a complex affair. If you are considering selling your practice, you would be wise to work with a qualified professional who has experience in valuing medical practices. You should know the value of your practice before you begin to negotiate a purchase price.

Current Trends in Practice Purchase Price

Most PPMCs state that they pay an average of five to eight times the projected earnings before interest and taxes (EBIT) of the practice for the next 12 months. In 1993, the average valuation multiples for physician groups were 0.8 times annual total revenues, 8.9 times EBIT, and $360,000 per physician.

By 1996, those valuation multiples had increased to 1.2 times annual revenues, 11.4 times EBIT, or $695,000 per physician. This increase can be attributed to greater competition for physician groups among PPMCs.

In a comparison of valuation multiples between single-specialty and multi-specialty group practices, single-specialty groups typically receive higher multiples of revenue, operating income, and per physician payouts because single-specialty groups tend to produce higher margins on their earnings and more revenues per physician. Since 1994, single-specialty valuation multiples have averaged 1.3 times annual revenue, 8.5 times operating income, and $940,000 per physician. Over the same period, multispecialty groups have average valuation multiples of 1.1 times annual revenue, 13.3 times operating income, and $440,000 per physician.

Trends in Acquisitions of Physician Groups

To conclude this chapter, we offer a brief overview of the PPMC marketplace and the level of acquisition activity occurring.

Practice Acquisition Trends

Oncology, ophthalmology, and occupational medicine are the most frequently acquired specialties. Two of those specialties, oncology and ophthalmology, have averaged the highest valuation multiples of any specialty since 1994. Oncology groups on average are valued at 1.4 times annual revenue, 9.5 times operating income, and $1,084,000 per physician. Ophthalmology valuations are not far behind, averaging 1.2 times annual revenue, 7.7 times operating income, and $1,035,000 per physician. Occupational medicine, a specialty with urgent or primary care characteristics, has averaged lower valuations, receiving 1.2 times annual revenues, 8.1 times operating income, and $784,000 per physician. Other specialties that are common acquisition targets include cardiology, radiology, emergency medicine, obstetrics/gynecology, and orthopedics. However, there have been too few announced acquisitions in these specialties to gather any relevant valuation data.

Level of Acquisition Activity

The number of publicly traded PPMCs has increased dramatically over the past few years, tripling since 1992 with 38 public PPMCs currently operating and at least two others, Omega Orthodontics and OrthAlliance, having recently filed to go public. A main growth strategy for all of these companies is to expand through acquisitions of group practices. The effect of this strategy can be seen in the increase of the number of publicly announced physician group transactions from 24 in 1993 to more than 200 in 1996.

As shown in Exhibit 4.3, from January 1994 through March 1997, 446 physician group transactions were publicly announced. This ranks second only to hospitals (462 transactions) as the most active of the health care segments. Both segments rank well ahead of home care, long-term care, and HMOs in terms of acquisition activity. The entire health care services industry ranks behind only business services as the most active industry in terms of total transactions in 1996, with 364 announced transactions.

Exhibit 4.3: Summary of Publicly Announced Health Care Transactions by Segment since January 1994

Segment	Number of Transactions
Hospitals	462
Medical groups	446
Home health	282
Long-term care	235
Lab/MRI/diagnostic	206
Rehabilitation	187
HMOs	150
Psychiatric	123
Other	305
Total	2,396

Source: Townsend Frew & Co. and Irving Levin & Associates; through March 31, 1997.

Exhibit 4.4 shows the most active physician group consolidators. MedPartners, Inc., and Physicians Resource Group have completed the most acquisitions to date with 43 each, followed by PhyCor, Inc., with 29.

Exhibit 4.4: The Most Acquisitive PPMCs, 1994–1996

PPMC	Number of Publicly Announced Transactions	Percent of Total Publicly Announced Transactions
1. MedPartners, Inc.*	43	9.5%
2. PhyCor, Inc.	29	6.4
3. Physicians Resource Group	43	9.5
4. OccuSystems, Inc.	23	5.1
5. American Oncology Resources, Inc.	29	6.4
6. EquiMed, Inc.	16	3.5
Total	183	40.4%

* Transaction totals include acquisitions by PPSI, Mullikin Medical, and Caremark.

Data from 1/1/94–12/31/96

5 Wall Street and Physician Practice Management Companies

Capital from Wall Street has fueled the development, reorganization, and growth of the PPMC industry in recent years. The significant infusion of capital has resulted in above-market returns on investment. This market dynamic is important for physicians considering affiliation with PPMCs where some of the purchase price consists of PPMC stock.

Wall Street has been willing to reward PPMCs by paying high valuation multiples. As explained in chapter 3, this multiple is also known as the price-to-earnings (P/E) ratio and is the price of a stock divided by its earnings per share (EPS). The higher the P/E ratio, the higher the premium placed on the company by the investment community. Therefore, the equity value on PPMC stocks is correlated to the projected EPS growth rate. Many investment banking firms employ research analysts who specialize in the health care or the PPMC industry. These analysts also consistently publish research reports on companies they follow and make recommendations to the investment community as to the future prospects of the company. They publish their estimates for future (usually two years) EPS of PPMCs (the average is known as the "street consensus"), which become the benchmark against which a company's performance is measured.

As a result of the over 30% returns on investment being generated by the industry, PPMCs have received significant attention from Wall Street. Other reasons for favorable treatment on Wall Street include the following:

- Size of market: The PPMC industry is estimated to generate expenditures of $250 billion.

- Demand: Observers predict that physicians will continue to require the resources offered by PPMCs to effectively manage the health care dollar.

- Fragmented industry: With only 5% of physicians affiliated with a PPMC and most physicians still practicing in a nongroup setting, observers predict dramatic consolidation activity.

- Economies of scale: Continued cost savings should be generated as groups consolidate infrastructure and realize purchasing economies.

PPMCs have performed better than most other segments in health care services because of the attractive growth and return characteristics. Exhibit 5.1 illustrates the differences in expected five-year growth in earnings of PPMCs versus HMOs, hospitals, and the pharmaceutical segments.

Exhibit 5.1: Five-Year EPS Growth, PPMC versus Other Health Care Segments

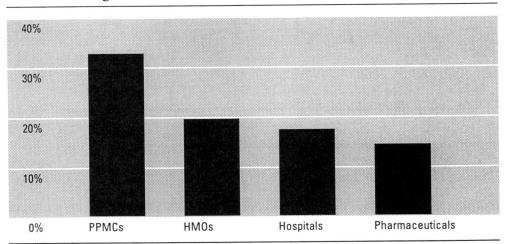

Likewise, PPMCs have higher price-to-earnings (P/E) ratios, on average, compared with other segments in the health care industry. Generally, investors apply a P/E commensurate with the projected earnings per share (EPS) growth rate. For example, if a company's EPS is projected to grow 20% during the next 12 months, and if investors have confidence that projected earnings will be met, the company may warrant a P/E of 20.0. Exhibit 5.2 contrasts the P/Es, based on 1997 EPS, of PPMCs and other publicly traded health care companies.

Exhibit 5.2: 1997 Estimated Price-to-Earning Multiples for
Selected Health Care Segments*

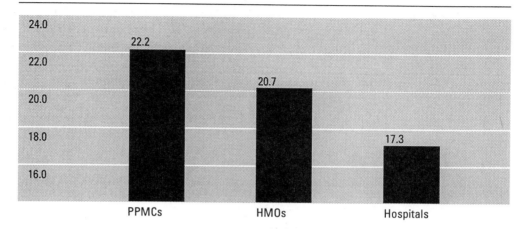

Note: Earnings estimates from I/B/E/S.

* Estimates as of 4/1/97. PPM companies include MedPartners, Inc., PhyCor Inc., Pediatrix Medical Group, OccuSystems Inc., Orthodontic Centers of American, FPA Medical Management, InPhyNet Medical Management, Physicians Resource Group, EmCare Holdings Inc, and American Oncology Resources Inc.

Other questions that investors ask when evaluating PPMCs include:

- Does the PPMC have dominant or major positions in its markets?

- Has the PPMC operated successfully in more than one market?

- Is the PPMC focused on developing its primary care network?

- Has the PPMC proved its ability to operate in a capitated market?

- Has the PPMC made adequate investments in information systems designed for a managed care environment?

- Does the PPMC have adequate access to capital to fund its future growth?

- Is the operational style "physician friendly" with strong leadership?

Wall Street also evaluates various financial performance measures to determine the appropriate equity value of a PPMC. Total revenues and market capitalization (equal to total shares outstanding times share price) also have a strong correlation to P/E ratios. The larger the revenues or equity value, the higher the valuation multiples. Publicly traded PPMCs, most of which have completed their initial public offering (IPO) within the last two years, have shown, on average, substantial increase in value since their IPO. Exhibit 5.3 highlights the returns that investors who invested in the initial offering have realized for selected PPMCs. We show those PPMCs that fared well in the upper portion and those that did not fare well because of earnings shortfalls in the lower portion.

Exhibit 5.3: IPO Aftermarket Performance

PPMC	Offering Price	Current Price (April 9, 1997)	Percent Change
PhyCor, Inc.	7.11	24.500	416.9%
FPA Medical Management	5.00	16.375	227.5
EmCare Holdings, Inc.	11.00	28.875	162.5
MedPartners	13.00	22.000	69.2
Pediatrix Medical Group	20.00	30.750	53.7
Complete Management, Inc.	9.00	11.750	30.6
Coastal Physician Group	11.50	1.750	84.8
Physician Reliance	9.75	5.625	42.3
American Oncology	10.50	8.500	19.0
Sheridan Healthcare	13.00	8.813	32.2

Note: Adjusted for stock splits.

Despite the success of many PPMCs, their stock values can be characterized by high volatility, which is often associated with high-growth segments. The following stock price chart illustrates the volatility of PPMCs versus the Standard & Poor (S&P) 500 since January 1, 1996 (see Exhibit 5.4).

Some PPMCs have been unable to meet Wall Street analysts' estimates, which typically results in a dramatic and immediate decline in the company's equity value. For example, on June 26, 1996, MedCath's share price fell 26% after it indicated to the market that its third-quarter EPS would fall short of analysts' estimates. Likewise, Physician Reliance Network's shares dropped nearly 50% on October 27, 1996, after its earnings fell short of expectations. Even when companies report results in line with estimates, Wall Street may penalize the stock price because of the higher standards it applies to stocks with high P/E ratios. For example, on October 21, 1996, PhyCor announced a 48% increase in its net income, in line with the street consensus. However, its stock declined 13% because of concerns relating to a possible slowdown in revenue growth and a slight decline in same-clinic growth.

Exhibit 5.4: Physician Practice Management Company Stock Index

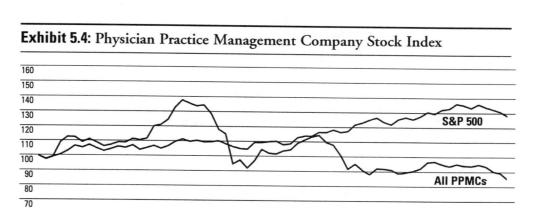

In evaluating an investment in a PPMC, or if considering accepting stock as part of a sale, physicians should dedicate significant time to researching the financial statement of the PPMC. Particular factors to evaluate or look for include the following.

- **Inflated P/E Ratio:** The average P/E ratio, based on 1997 estimated EPS, is 22.2, versus 17.3 for the S&P 500; as the PPMC market matures, P/E ratios will come more in line with the overall market, and valuations will decline commensurably.

- **Future Earnings Largely Dependent on Acquisitions:** PPMCs that are expected to meet earnings growth rates that exceed the growth of the underlying business of the PPMC will be forced to acquire groups in order to show higher earnings; such pressure can lead to the pursuit and closure of transactions that are not in the best long-term interests of the PPMC.

- **Deterioration of "Quality of Earnings":** PPMCs may resort to adjustments in reserves, or other "one-time" adjustments that artificially inflate net income in order to meet Wall Street EPS estimates.

- **Unfocused Business Strategy:** In order to realize operational synergies, PPMCs must remain focused on markets, services, and specialties that are consistent with core competencies.

- **Operational "Value Addeds" Not Apparent:** PPMCs that are unable to demonstrate operational efficiencies, such as "same clinic" growth, will have a difficult time attracting acquisition candidates over the long term.

Conclusion

As physicians and physician groups consider PPMC affiliation, they will need to carefully consider the multitude of factors that have been outlined in this book. The better informed the physician on all these aspects, including the view of PPMCs from Wall Street, the more likely the decision whether to affiliate will be the right one.

Appendix
Public Physician Practice Management Companies

Advanced Health Corporation (Nasdaq: ADVH)

Advanced Health Corp. vertically integrates practice and network management services with clinical information systems. The management services provided by the company include physician practice and network development, marketing, payor contracting, financial and administrative management, clinical information management, human resource management, and practice and network governance. The company also provides clinical information systems through its Med-E-Systems subsidiary that give physicians patient-specific clinical and health plan information at the point of care. As of June 1997, the company provides practice and network management and consulting services to over 1,800 physicians.

Quick Facts[1]

Specialty:	Multispecialty/Primary Care
IPO Date:	October 1996
Chairman/CEO:	Jon Edelson, MD
Headquarters:	Tarrytown, NY

Recent Acquisitions

6/17/97—Advanced Health Corp. signed a long-term network management contract with Assured Care Network Management Company in Chattanooga, Tennessee. Assured Care Network Management Company is related to Assured Care of Chattanooga, an IPA with 486 physicians and 186 clinical sites in the Chattanooga area. Terms were not disclosed. *6/10/97*—Advanced Health Corp. signed a long-term practice management agreement with Bergen Medical Alliance, P.A., a seven-physician multispecialty group in Bergen, New Jersey. *6/2/97–2/24/97*—Advanced Health Corp. signed a contract to merge Millennium Medical, P.A. and Genesis Medical, P.C., two physician groups in northern New Jersey. Millennium Medical, a practice managed by Advanced Health since September 1996, is based in Union County, New Jersey, and is a primary care-based multispecialty group with 10 physicians. Genesis Medical, based in Cranford, New Jersey,

---

1. See Table A.-1 at the end of this appendix for shares outstanding, market capitalization, last 12 months revenue, and last 12 months net income statistics for the practice management companies described in Appendix A.

is a primary care-driven group composed of 13 physicians. The merger creates a 23-doctor, fully integrated group with multiple care centers in the community.

American Oncology Resources, Inc. (Nasdaq: AORI)

American Oncology Resources, Inc., is a national physician practice management company that focuses exclusively on oncology. The company provides comprehensive management services under long-term agreements to 256 physicians practicing in 23 groups in 15 states. Many of those practices provide a broad range of medical services to cancer patients, integrating the specialties of medical oncology, radiation oncology, and hematology.

Quick Facts

Specialty:	Oncology
IPO Date:	June 1995
Chairman/CEO:	R. Dale Ross
Headquarters:	Houston, TX

Recent Acquisitions

4/3/97—American Oncology Resources added 23 new oncologists during the first quarter of 1997, bringing its total oncologists to 250. Ten were added in Virginia, four in Indiana, and nine in various other locations.

Coastal Physician Group, Inc. (NYSE: DR)

Coastal Physician Group is a physician practice management company that provides a broad range of health care and administrative services to physicians, hospitals, government agencies, managed care programs, employers, and other health care organizations nationwide. The company provides these services in more than 530 settings, of which more than 500 include physician, hospital, and government contracts and include 32 primary care practices.

Quick Facts

Specialty:	Hospital Based
IPO Date:	June 1991
Chairman/CEO:	Steven Scott, MD
Headquarters:	Durham, NC

Recent Acquisitions

12/3/96—Coastal completed the previously announced sale of HealthNet, its New Jersey-based clinic operations, to the Valley Care Corp., the parent of Valley Hospital. Coastal realized $9 million in cash proceeds from the transaction, which it will use to reduce indebtedness. HealthNet employs 32 physicians at the group's nine primary care sites in New York and New Jersey. The Valley Hospital is a 421-bed acute care facility based in

Ridgewood, New Jersey. **11/25/96**—Coastal completed the previously announced sale of MedCost, Inc., a preferred provider organization, to a joint venture between North Carolina Baptist Hospital and Carolinas HealthCare System. Coastal realized approximately $14 million in cash proceeds from the transaction.

Complete Management, Inc. (ASE: CMI)

Complete Management, Inc., offers a broad range of management and support services for medical practice groups and hospitals in the greater New York metropolitan and Tri-State area. The company provides full management services to 150 physicians and billing and collection services to approximately 9,000 physicians.

Quick Facts

Specialty:	Multispecialty/Primary Care
IPO Date:	December 1995
Chairman/CEO:	Steven Rabinovci
Headquarters:	New York, NY

Recent Acquisitions

6/17/97—Complete Management purchased Consumer Health Network, Inc., the largest PPO in the state of New Jersey, for $12 million, consisting of $8 million in cash and $4 million in stock. Consumer Health Network has recently expanded into New York and Connecticut. Its network consists of approximately 7,800 physicians and 120 hospitals, serving 975,000 lives. **6/5/97**—Complete Management announced that it completed three transactions to manage medical practices with a total of eight primary care physicians, consisting of seven OB/GYN doctors and one family practice doctor. The practices are located Westchester County, New York. The transactions were arranged and financed on behalf of its client, Northern Metropolitan Medical, P.C. **3/17/97**—Complete Management, Inc., ended plans to acquire Amedisys, Inc., because neither side could agree on terms, including price. The two companies first announced the planned transaction in October 1996, when Complete Management said it offered $36.8 million to $41.9 million in stock for Amedisys, a provider of home health care, medical staffing, and outpatient surgery services based in Baton Rouge, Louisiana.

EmCare Holdings, Inc. (Nasdaq: EMCR)

EmCare Holdings, Inc., is a leading provider of physician practice management services in hospital emergency room departments and other practice settings. The company has managed emergency physician practices for more than 20 years, primarily in hospitals with higher volume emergency departments. The company recruits physicians, evaluates their credentials, arranges contracts, and schedules their services. EmCare assists in such operational areas as staff coordination, quality assurances, and departmental accreditation, and provides billing, recordkeeping, third-party payment programs, and other administrative services. As of March 1997, the company had management contracts relating to 143 emergency departments in 19 states with approximately 2.6 million patient visits per year.

Quick Facts

Specialty:	Hospital Based
IPO Date:	December 1994
Chairman/CEO:	Leonard M. Riggs, Jr, MD
Headquarters:	Dallas, TX

Recent Acquisitions

5/7/97—EmCare Holdings announced definitive agreements to acquire three emergency physician practices in Georgia. These contracts will provide emergency physician practice management services to four facilities and generate revenues of $7.7 million and 111,000 patient visits. 1/8/97—EmCare Holdings acquired the Gould Group, Inc., a physician practice management company operating 41 emergency departments throughout rural areas in Florida, Oklahoma, Louisiana, Texas, Arkansas, and Mississippi. The Gould Group generated approximately $15 million in 1995 revenue.

EquiMed, Inc. (Nasdaq: EQMD)

EquiMed, Inc., is a national physician practice management company that provides oncology services through its networks of specialty medical providers. As of May 1997, the company owns, operates, or manages 39 radiation oncology centers. Additionally, EquiMed currently manages five complementary subspecialty medical practices in medical oncology, urology, and internal medicine. Effective November 1, 1996, EquiMed sold its ophthalmology operations to Physicians Resource Group for $55.1 million in cash and the assumption by PRG of approximately $16.6 million of liabilities.

Quick Facts

Specialty:	Oncology
IPO Date:	November 1993
Chairman/CEO:	Douglas R. Colkitt, MD
Headquarters:	State College, PA

Recent Acquisitions

5/19/97—EquiMed announced the finalization of the acquisitions of several companies from Douglas Colkitt, MD. EquiMed announced the acquisitions on February 12, 1997. The acquisitions include Russell Data Services, Inc., Trident International Accounting, Inc., Billing Services, Inc., Trident International Accounting, Inc., Billing Services International, Inc., Tiger Communications International, LTD, and an 80% interest in Tiger Services Private Limited. These companies are engaged in a variety of businesses providing outsourcing for accounting, billing, data processing, collections, and other administrative services. Total consideration paid to the companies was $6 million in cash plus a potential earnout of up to $9.3 million in EquiMed common stock. **5/1/97—**

EquiMed acquired the practice of Dr. Joseph Won in Detroit, Michigan, and Dr. Madhu Mohan in Washington, DC. Total consideration for the practices was $4.4 million, consisting of $3.3 million in cash and $1.1 million in notes payable. The acquisition brings the total number of EquiMed medical and radiation oncology centers to 39.

FPA Medical Management, Inc. (Nasdaq: FPAM)

FPA Medical Management, Inc., is a national health care management services organization that organizes and manages primary care physician practices and networks that contract with HMOs and other prepaid health insurance plans to provide physician and related health care services to payor members who select FPA primary care physicians. FPA also assumes administrative functions necessary in a managed care environment related to claims adjudication, utilization management of medical services, payor contract negotiations, and the operation of management information systems. As of June 6, 1997, FPA is affiliated with 23,100 physicians in 27 states.

Quick Facts

Specialty:	Multispecialty/Primary Care
IPO Date:	October 1994
Chairman/CEO:	Seth Flam, MD—President and CEO
	Sol Lizerbram, MD—Chairman
Headquarters:	San Diego, CA

Recent Acquisitions

6/6/97—FPA Medical Management agreed to buy HealthCap, Inc., for $48 million in stock. HealthCap, located in San Diego, develops and manages primary care and women's health medical groups and OB/GYN and multispecialty physician equity model networks. The acquisition will add 2,100 doctors in California, Florida, Georgia, Nevada, and Missouri, and $55 million in revenue to FPA's operations. **3/17/97**—FPA completed its acquisition of AHI Healthcare Systems, Inc. for $117 million in stock. FPA will pay 0.391 share of its stock for each of AHI's 14.6 million outstanding shares. The transaction forms a company with approximately $1 billion in revenue that provides services to more than 800,000 managed health care plan members in 25 states.

Integrated Orthopaedics, Inc. (ASE: IOI) (Formerly DRCA Medical)

Integrated Orthopaedics, Inc., specializes in the management of orthopedic medicine practices and other musculoskeletal-related patient services. As of December 31, 1996, Integrated Orthopaedics managed a musculoskeletal-related health care delivery system in Houston, Texas, which included an orthopedic medicine practice, three work hardening clinics, two physical/occupational therapy centers, and one magnetic resonance imaging center.

Quick Facts

Specialty:	Orthopedics
IPO Date:	NA
Chairman/CEO:	Jose E. Kauachi
Headquarters:	Houston, TX

Recent Acquisitions

5/15/97—Integrated Orthopaedics announced that it has initiated affiliation discussions with 200 orthopedic specialists in nine states. 1/6/97—Integrated Orthopaedics sold its occupational medicine business to OccuSystems, Inc., for $7.6 million. The transaction included four occupational medicine centers in Houston and three facilities in Little Rock, Arkansas. Also included in the transaction was a mobile testing service based in Houston.

MedCath, Inc. (Nasdaq: MCTH)

MedCath provides cardiology and cardiovascular services through the development, operation, and management of heart hospitals and other specialized cardiac care facilities and provides physician practice management services. The company affiliates with leading cardiologists and cardiovascular and vascular surgeons in targeted geographical markets. The company's strategy is to establish and maintain localized, fully-integrated networks that will provide quality, cost-effective diagnosis and treatment of cardiovascular disease.

Quick Facts

Specialty:	Cardiology
IPO Date:	December 1994
Chairman/CEO:	Stephen R. Puckett
Headquarters:	Charlotte, NC

Recent Acquisitions

5/16/97—MedCath acquired Los Angeles, California-based Ultimed, Inc., which provides cardiovascular disease management services to IPAs, HMOs, and large cardiology groups. Ultimed currently manages more than 150,000 capitated and noncapitated lives. Terms of the transaction were not disclosed.

Medical Asset Management, Inc. (Nasdaq: MAMT)

Medical Asset Management, Inc., is a physician practice management company which develops contractual affiliations with physician practices that provide for management by the company and clinical autonomy for the physicians. Through its subsidiary, Healthcare Professional Management, Inc., the company also offers a full array of management services to affiliated physicians and other independent health care entities under long-term service contracts as a management service organization. At the end of 1996, the company had equity affiliations with 28 physician practices having a total of 48 physicians.

Quick Facts

Specialty:	Multispecialty/Primary Care
IPO Date:	June 1994
Chairman/CEO:	John Regan
Headquarters:	Mesa, AZ

Recent Acquisitions

5/8/97—Medical Asset Management announced that since the beginning of 1997, it has affiliated with eight physician practices involving 12 physicians in six states. Additionally, the company has agreements with 10 additional practices involving 13 physicians in six states. **12/23/96**—Medical Asset Management entered into a long-term management agreement with Pediatric Alliance, P.C., a general pediatric practice located in Pittsburgh, Pennsylvania, which includes 37 physicians in 14 care centers.

MedPartners, Inc. (NYSE: MDM)

MedPartners, Inc., develops, consolidates, and manages health care delivery systems. Through the company's network of affiliated group and IPA physicians, MedPartners provides primary and specialty health care services to prepaid enrollees and fee-for-service patients. Including its acquisition of InPhyNet Medical Management, Inc., and Aetna U.S. Healthcare's physician management business, MedPartners will operate physician practices in 36 states. At that time it will be affiliated with 12,312 physicians, including 2,945 in group practices, 6,917 through IPA relationships, and 2,450 hospital-based physicians. MedPartners' prescription benefit management division fills over 50 million prescriptions annually.

Quick Facts

Specialty:	Multispecialty/Primary Care
IPO Date:	February 1995
Chairman/CEO:	Larry R. House
Headquarters:	Birmingham, AL

Recent Acquisitions

5/21/97—MedPartners, Inc., lowered the price it will pay for InPhyNet Medical Management, Inc., by about 10% to $377.5 million after InPhyNet restated its earnings for 1996 and the first quarter of 1997. MedPartners will now exchange 1.18 shares for each of InPhyNet's 16.7 million shares outstanding, instead of the 1.31 announced in the original January 20 agreement. 5/20/97— MedPartners acquired 172-physician Piedmont IPA in Durham, North Carolina. The network includes 60 primary care and 116 specialty providers. Piedmont IPA is responsible for the medical needs of 2,275 prepaid lives as well as fee-for-service patients. After the acquisition, MedPartners-affiliated physicians provide care for more than 32,000 prepaid covered lives in North Carolina. 5/2/97—MedPartners completed the purchase of Aetna U.S. Healthcare's physician management business and family medical centers. Terms of the acquisition of Aetna Professional Management Corp., Healthways Family Medical Centers, and affiliated group practices were not disclosed. Analysts have estimated the price at $50 million to $80 million.

Pediatrix Medical Group, Inc. (NYSE: PDX)

Pediatrix is the nation's largest provider of physician management services to hospital-based neonatal intensive care units (NICUs). As of May 31, the company provides services to 82 NICUs, eight pediatric intensive care units, and three pediatrics departments in 20 states and Puerto Rico and employs or contracts with approximately 230 physicians.

Quick Facts

Specialty:	Hospital Based
IPO Date:	September 1995
Chairman/CEO:	Roger J. Medel, MD
Headquarters:	Ft. Lauderdale, FL

Recent Acquisitions

5/29/97—Pediatrix announced the cash acquisition of Carolina Neonatology Associates, P.A., which operates a neonatal intensive care unit in Columbia, South Carolina. In 1996, the unit generated 5,000 patient days. The acquisition is Pediatrix' second in South Carolina. 4/21/97— Pediatrix completed the acquisition of Foothill Medical Group, Inc., a Pasadena, California-based neonatology physician group practice that operates two neonatal intensive care units. The Foothill practice generated 12,000 patient days during 1996. It is Pediatrix' third group practice acquisition in the Southern California market in less than two years. 3/27/97—Pediatrix acquired NeoFirst, Inc., P.C., a neonatology physician group practice that operates two neonatal intensive care units in South Bend, Indiana. The transaction was Pediatrix' first in Indiana. 3/20/97— Pediatrix acquired Tacoma, Washington-based Neonatal Associates, Inc. The group practice provides services to two Tacoma-area neonatal intensive care units and generated approximately 15,000 patient days during 1996. The transaction marks Pediatrix' entry into the state of Washington.

PhyCor, Inc. (Nasdaq: PHYC)

PhyCor, Inc., acquires and operates multispecialty medical clinics and develops and manages IPAs. As of May 1997, PhyCor operated 48 clinics with approximately 3,280 physicians in 28 states and manages IPAs with over 15,800 physicians in 23 markets. PhyCor intends to position its affiliated clinics and IPAs to be the physician component of integrated health care systems. PhyCor seeks to acquire primary care-oriented multispecialty clinics that have significant market share. After acquiring a clinic, PhyCor expands its operations by adding physicians, developing managed care relationships, and expanding ancillary services.

Quick Facts

Specialty:	Multispecialty/Primary Care
IPO Date:	January 1992
Chairman/CEO:	Joseph C. Hutts
Headquarters:	Nashville, TN

Recent Acquisitions

5/1/97—PhyCor, Inc., completed its acquisition of Greater Chesapeake Medical Group, a 28-physician multispecialty clinic in Annapolis, Maryland. Other terms were not disclosed. The acquisition marks PhyCor's entry to the Maryland market. **2/28/97**— PhyCor affiliated with an additional 95 physicians in transactions with the St. Petersburg Medical Clinic and Suncoast Medical Clinic, multispecialty clinics in St. Petersburg, Florida, and has entered a long-term service agreement with the newly formed St. Petersburg-Suncoast Medical Group. Other terms were not disclosed. **2/25/97**—PhyCor completed its acquisition of Vancouver Clinic, a 66-physician multispecialty group in Vancouver, Washington. Other terms were not disclosed.

PhyMatrix Corporation (Nasdaq: PHMX)

PhyMatrix Corp. provides management and related medical support services to disease specialty and primary care physicians. The company's primary strategy is to develop specialty care networks in specific geographic locations by affiliating with disease specialty and primary care physicians. Since its first acquisition in 1994, the company has acquired the practices of and affiliated with 130 physicians and acquired several medical support services companies.

Quick Facts

Specialty:	Multispecialty/Primary Care
IPO Date:	January 1996
Chairman/CEO:	Abraham D. Gosman
Headquarters:	West Palm Beach, FL

Recent Acquisitions

6/12/97—PhyMatrix Corp. acquired two diagnostic imaging centers in Dade County, Florida, for approximately $9.1 million in stock. PhyMatrix also announced that it had entered into a management agreement for a radiation therapy center in New York. The base management fee to PhyMatrix is approximately $400,000 per year. 4/7/97—PhyMatrix acquired Breathco, Inc., a specialty physician network company that provides pulmonary physician network services through 100 physician providers to over 400,000 covered lives in South Florida.

Physician Reliance Network, Inc. (Nasdaq: PHYN)

Physician Reliance Network, Inc., provides professional management services to physician groups that diagnose and treat cancer. As of March 31, 1997, the company managed the practices of 310 physicians in 108 locations, including 17 cancer centers. Physician Reliance Network provides the management, facilities, administrative and technical support, and ancillary services necessary for physicians to establish and maintain a fully integrated network of outpatient oncology care.

Quick Facts

Specialty:	Oncology
IPO Date:	November 1994
Chairman/CEO:	Merrick H. Reese, MD
Headquarters:	Dallas, TX

Recent Acquisitions

4/29/97—Physician Reliance Network announced that it had affiliated with 51 medical oncologists, three radiation oncologists, two gynecological oncologists, and eight other physicians during the first quarter of 1997. Other terms were not disclosed. Additionally, the company announced that it had entered a service agreement with a group of seven medical oncologists located in Seattle, Washington, effective April 1, 1997.

Physicians Resource Group, Inc. (NYSE: PRG)

Physicians Resource Group, Inc., provides practice management services to ophthalmic and optometric practices. PRG develops integrated eye care delivery systems through affiliations with locally prominent eye care practices in selected geographic markets. PRG acquires the operating assets of these practices and develops the practices into comprehensive eye care networks by providing management expertise, marketing, information systems, capital resources, and ancillary services, such as surgery centers and optical dispensaries. As of January 9, 1997, the company had operations in 25 states.

Quick Facts

Specialty:	Ophthalmology
IPO Date:	June 1995
Chairman/CEO:	Emmit E. Moore
Headquarters:	Dallas, TX

Recent Acquisitions

5/14/97—Physicians Resource Group announced that it has made seven eye care practice acquisitions in New York, Kentucky, Florida, Ohio, and Texas, which included nine ophthalmologists, nine optometrists, 18 locations, and 10 optical shops. These eye care acquisitions required cash of $6.4 million and $3.4 million of 7% convertible notes.

1/9/97— Physicians Resource Group announced that it had completed the acquisition of the assets of eight separate eye care practices since the beginning of December. Five of the practices are located in the Dallas, San Antonio and Houston, Texas, markets; the remainder are located in Chicago, Illinois; Orlando, Florida; and Roanoke Rapids, North Carolina. Total consideration for the practices was $10.3 million, consisting of $680,000 cash and PRG stock worth $9.6 million. The eight practices combined have 14 ophthalmologists and five optometrists at 16 locations and operate six optical dispensaries.

11/22/96—Physicians Resource Group closed its acquisition of American Ophthalmic, Inc. (AOI). The purchase price for the acquisition was approximately $59.0 million, consisting of $30.9 million cash and PRG stock valued at $28.1 million. AOI shareholders may receive an additional $8.2 million in April 1997 if certain eye care practices in AOI's acquisition pipeline agree to be acquired by PRG. PRG also retired approximately $44.5 million and assumed approximately $13.7 million in AOI indebtedness.

Physicians' Specialty Corporation (Nasdaq: ENTS)

Physicians' Specialty Corp. provides physician practice management services to physician practices and health care providers specializing in the treatment and management of diseases and disorders of the ear, nose, and throat, and head and neck. The company's primary objective is to develop, manage, and integrate ENT physician and related specialty practices which will provide quality cost-effective medical and surgical services to fee-for-service patients and capitated managed care enrollees. After the company's initial public offering on March 26, 1997, it was affiliated with 23 physicians, one dentist, and 26 allied health care professionals operating in 19 clinical locations in Georgia and Alabama.

Quick Facts

Specialty:	Ear, nose, and throat, and head and neck (ENT)
IPO Date:	March 1997
Chairman/President:	Ramie A. Tritt, MD
Headquarters:	Atlanta, GA

Recent Acquisitions

3/20/97—Concurrent with its public offering, Physicians' Specialty Corp. acquired Atlanta ENT, Metropolitan Ear, Nose & Throat P.C., Atlanta Head and Neck Surgery, P.C., and Ear, Nose & Throat Associates, P.C., which are all located in Atlanta, and W.J. Cornay, III, MD, P.C., which is located in Birmingham, Alabama. Total consideration for the practices was $17.1 million.

ProMedCo Management Company (Nasdaq: PMCO)

ProMedCo consolidates its affiliated physician groups into primary-care driven multispecialty networks. The company focuses on pre-managed care secondary markets located principally outside of or adjacent to large metropolitan areas. ProMedCo commenced operations in December 1994 and as of June 1997 was affiliated with 183 physicians in Texas, Nevada, Alabama, Florida, Kentucky, New Hampshire, and Maine.

Quick Facts

Specialty:	Multispecialty/Primary Care
IPO Date:	March 1997
Chairman/CEO:	Richard E. Ragsdale
Headquarters:	Ft. Worth, TX

Recent Acquisitions

6/10/97—ProMedCo signed a letter of intent to acquire Portland, Maine-based Health Plans, Inc., which provides capitation management services through risk contracting with third-party payors. Health Plans, Inc., provides services that cover approximately 30,000 capitated lives, and it manages a network of 240 physicians and several hospitals in the Maine and New Hampshire area. 5/1/97—ProMedCo announced that it completed its affiliation with Naples Medical Center, P.A., a 36-physician multispecialty group in Naples, Florida. Other terms were not disclosed.

Response Oncology, Inc. (Nasdaq: ROIX)

Response Oncology is a comprehensive cancer management company. It owns and/or operates a network of outpatient treatment centers that provide stem cell-supported high dose chemotherapy and cancer treatment services; owns the assets of and manages the business aspects of oncology practices; and conducts clinical cancer research on behalf of pharmaceutical manufacturers. As of June 1997, about 350 oncologists were affiliated with the company.

Quick Facts

Specialty:	Oncology
IPO Date:	April 1987
President/CEO:	Joseph T. Clark
Headquarters:	Memphis, TN

Recent Acquisitions

12/2/96—Response Oncology announced that it acquired the nonmedical assets of the practices of Drs. Haraf, Antonucci, McCormack & Kerns general partnership located in Knoxville, Tennessee, and Weinreb, Weisburg & Weiss, P.A., located in Tamarac, Florida.

Sheridan Healthcare, Inc. (Nasdaq: SHCR)

Sheridan Healthcare provides specialist physician services at hospitals and ambulatory surgical facilities in the areas of anesthesia, neonatology, pediatrics, emergency services, and obstetrics. The company also owns and operates, or manages, office-based primary care and obstetrical physician practices. As of April 1997, Sheridan was affiliated with more than 200 physicians practicing under 43 specialty contracts at 27 hospitals and 18 office locations.

Quick Facts

Specialty:	Hospital Based
IPO Date:	October 1995
Chairman/CEO:	Mitchell Eisenburg, MD
Headquarters:	Hollywood, FL

Recent Acquisitions

4/11/97—Sheridan Healthcare completed the sale of its rheumatology practices, which consist of six rheumatologists practicing in four office locations, to Continucare Corporation for $3.3 million in cash. Sheridan does not expect to realize a significant gain or loss on the transaction. 1/3/97—Sheridan Healthcare said it will sell 11 office-based physician practices in Florida, resulting in a fourth-quarter pre-tax charge of approximately $17 million. Terms were not disclosed. Sheridan said it had already completed the sale of one of the practices located in the Miami/Ft. Lauderdale area. The sale is part of Sheridan's plan to focus on its hospital-based business and its obstetric practices.

Specialty Care Network, Inc. (Nasdaq: SCNI)

Specialty Care Network focuses on musculoskeletal disease management. It seeks to affiliate with leading musculoskeletal practices in targeted markets, manage and expand its affiliated practices, and develop integrated regional musculoskeletal around its affiliated practices. As of April 1997, the company managed nine practices located in Florida, Georgia, Maryland, New Jersey, and Pennsylvania. It also managed one outpatient surgery center and one outpatient magnetic resonance imaging center owned by two of its affiliated practices.

Quick Facts

Specialty:	Orthopedics
IPO Date:	February 1997
President/CEO:	Kerry R. Hicks—CEO
Headquarters:	Lakewood, CO

Recent Acquisitions

4/4/97—Specialty Care Network affiliated with The Orthopedics and Sports Medicine Center II, P.A., a nine-physician practice in Annapolis, Maryland. 3/1/97—During March, Specialty Care Network acquired three single physician practices in Florida, Maryland, and Georgia. Total consideration was $135,000 in cash and approximately $4 million in stock.

Table A.1: Public PPMC Financial Data

Numbers in thousands; market capitalization as of 6/17/97.

	Shares Outstanding	Market Capitalization	Last 12 Months Revenue	Last 12 Months Net Income	Last 12 Months as of	Notes:
Advanced Health Corp.—ADVH	7,235	$124,357	$25,451	$396	03/31	
American Oncology Resources—AORI	28,646	$411,784	$308,006	$18,275	03/31	
Coastal Physician Group—DR	24,384	$45,720	$524,089	($169,908)	03/31	Results exclude $40.3 million gain on sale of assets.
Complete Management, Inc.—CMI	10,050	$127,515	$40,808	$6,017	03/31	
EmCare Holdings—EMCR	8,187	$268,121	$211,532	$11,174	03/31	Results exclude $8.5 million in fines related to a lawsuit settlement.
EquiMed, Inc.—EQMD	27,734	$107,469	$56,865	$5,275	12/31	Pro forma for sale of ophthalmology operations to PRG 11/1/96. Results exclude $212,000 loss on early extinguishment of debt.
FPA Medical Management, Inc.—FPAM	30,868	$667,515	$801,964	($65,505)	03/31	Results exclude $36.8 million in merger and restructuring charges.
Integrated Orthopaedics—IOI	5,287	$27,755	$6,254	($2,545)	03/31	Results exclude a $415,000 gain from restructuring. Last 12 months results are estimated by annualizing first quarter 1997 results. IOI sold its occupational health business to OccuSystems effective 12/31/96, and no year-end pro forma numbers were available.
MedCath, Inc.—MCTH	11,153	$169,520	$87,262	$6,525	03/31	
Medical Asset Management, Inc.—MAMT	13,473	$36,210	$23,908	$1,967	12/31	
MedPartners, Inc.—MDM	171,518	$3,902,039	$4,995,958	$109,183	03/31	Results exclude $274.2 million in merger expenses.
Pediatrix Medical Group—PDX	14,916	$678,667	$91,719	$14,816	03/31	
PhyCor, Inc.—PHYC	63,495	$2,182,628	$1,701,913	$40,997	03/31	
PhyMatrix Corp.—PHMX	22,978	$356,155	$,222,911	$13,691	04/30	
Physician Reliance Network—PHYN	48,295	$516,154	$339,779	$20,114	03/31	
Physicians Resource Group—PRG	29,977	$281,034	$346,872	$17,292	03/31	Results exclude $3 million in merger costs and $890,000 in patent litigation defense costs.
Physicians' Specialty Corp.—ENTS	5,905	$39,118	$22,775	$2,266	03/31	The company was not operational in first quarter 1996. Last 12 months results are 1996 year-end numbers plus first quarter 1997 results.
ProMedCo Management Co.—PMCO	8,784	$76,859	$78,020	$1,391	03/31	Results exclude $682,000 in merger costs.
Response Oncology, Inc.—ROIX	11,968	$83,773	$78,629	$1,866	03/31	Results exclude $608,000 in nonrecurring financing costs.
Sheridan Healthcare—SHCR	6,715	$73,861	$95,818	$3,248	03/31	Results exclude a $17.4 million write-down of office-based net assets and a $225,000 loss on terminated contracts.
Specialty Care Network, Inc.—SCNI	15,059	$161,886	$40,808	$4,474	03/31	

B Appendix
Private Physician Practice Management Companies

Arcon HealthCare

The Arcon HealthCare system was designed to improve the range and quality of medical services to local residents. Arcon HealthCare is supplanting fragmented care for citizens outside America's big cities with access to essential services in their home towns. As local markets dictate, Arcon will contract with specialists, hospitals, and a full spectrum of allied and related service partners to create a community-based delivery system. Arcon's provider network will include high-quality local physicians as well as specialists from nearby urban markets who may already be serving some of the community's health care needs. This delivery system will apply the same state-of-the-art, quality managed care principles and techniques found in the best urban programs to facilitate broader access to essential, specialty, ancillary, and urgent care.

4/24/97—Arcon HealthCare announced that it plans to build a $6 million, 20,000-square-foot center that will provide 24-hour emergency care, outpatient surgery, and diagnostic services to 20,000 people in Pflugerville, Texas.

1/27/97—Arcon HealthCare entered into a long-term agreement to operate the Pahrump Medical Center in Pahrump, Nevada, which is 63 miles northwest of Las Vegas. The two-year contract includes an option to purchase the facility and two possible 50-year extensions.

Quick Facts
President: Hud Connery, Jr
Headquarters: Nashville, TN

Cornerstone Physicians Corp.

Cornerstone is a privately held physician practice management company headquartered in Irvine, California. In addition to use of the traditional equity model, Cornerstone, founded in 1994, also offers physician practice management services and consultation without an ownership transaction. Cornerstone operates regional offices from Atlanta, Georgia; Irvine, California; Roanoke, Virginia; Rochester, New York; Dallas, Texas; and

Pittsburgh, Pennsylvania. It targets primary care practices in markets where the managed care penetration rate is between 15% and 20%.

Cornerstone operates a total of three clinics in two states with 66 affiliated or managed physicians. The majority of the equity is held by the founder, participating physicians, and senior management team. The balance is owned by InterWest Partners (Menlo Park, CA), Crosspoint Venture Partners (Lost Altos, CA), and Accel Partners (Embarcadero, CA)—the Company's capital venture partners. The company plans to make a public offering in 1997.

Quick Facts

Specialty:	Multispecialty/Primary Care
CEO:	John Seitz
Headquarters:	Irvine, CA

First Physician Care

First Physician Care, headquartered in Atlanta, Georgia, is a multiregional physician practice management company that develops, manages, and operates primary care-focused medical group practices and independent practice associations. Managed care payors access FPC's delivery systems through its affiliated physician-led medical groups, IPAs, administrative and medical management services, information technology, and capital to its physicians through various partnership structures.

FPC serves over 200 physician partners in 49 clinic sites under its medical group operations and is affiliated with an additional 1,000 physicians through its IPA management subsidiary Precept Healthcare Group. FPC operates in six states. Two of the nation's leading health care investors, Welsh, Carson, Anderson & Stowe and The Sprout Group have invested over $30 million in First Physician Care.

1/10/97—First Physician Care merged with Physician Capital Partners, which provides management services for Health Partners Medical Group of Fort Worth, Texas. Health Partners adds 83 providers, including 69 family practitioners, and 45,000 commercial-equivalent HMO lives to FPC's operations. Terms were not disclosed.

8/1/96—First Physician Care entered the Midwest with the completion of its acquisition of Riverbend Physicians & Surgeons, a 20-provider multispecialty clinic located in the St. Louis metropolitan area.

Quick Facts

Specialty:	Multispecialty/Primary Care
President:	Stephen A. George, MD
Headquarters:	Atlanta, GA

GynCor, Inc.

GynCor, Inc., provides comprehensive management and clinical support services to integrated networks of physicians specializing in the field of reproductive medicine, primarily subspecialties of obstetrics and gynecology. The company currently manages an integrated network of 25 fertility clinics and has $50 million in revenue. GynCor filed for a $25 million initial public offering in July 1996 but decided to postpone the offering when several publicly traded PPMCs reported lower-than-expected earnings, causing prices in the sector to fall. GynCor plans to make the offering when it reaches $100 million in annual revenue.

HealthCap, Inc.

HealthCap, Inc., is a physician practice management company based in San Diego, founded in 1992 by C. Michael Wright, MD. HealthCap is dedicated to the development of medical groups and physician-centered managed care providers as flexible, financially viable alternatives to HMOs and hospital-based health care systems. As of June 1997, HealthCap was affiliated with 2,100 doctors in California, Florida, Georgia, Nevada, and Missouri and provided services to over 325,000 capitated HMO enrollees. On June 6, 1997, the company announced it would be acquired by FPA Medical Management (Nasdaq: FPAM) for $48 million in stock.

2/17/97—HealthCap entered a practice management agreement with Southeast Women's Healthcare, a 350-physician OB/GYN network serving South Florida's tri-county area that provides medical services to approximately 100,000 patients.

2/13/97—HealthCap agreed to provide management services to Gateway Physicians Network, an 85-physician IPA providing services to 15,000 St. Louis residents. Prior to its agreement with HealthCap, Gateway Physicians was managed by a subsidiary of the Barnes Jewish Christian hospital network in St. Louis.

Quick Facts

Specialty:	Primary Care and OB/GYN
Chairman:	C. Michael Wright, MD
Headquarters:	San Diego, CA

Health Partners, Inc.

Health Partners, Inc., focuses on the acquisition of primary care-oriented multispecialty clinics and is affiliated with 1,021 physicians through its owned groups and IPAs. The company has physician group practice and network management affiliations in Northern Virginia, Ohio, New York, Texas, and Washington, DC. Health Partners is jointly owned by Oxford Health Plans, WellPoint Health Network, and other individual investors. Its annual revenue is $146 million, of which 80% comes from clinics with full professional capitation. The company received $15 million in capital from Oxford as of year-end 1995 and has commitments to receive up to $50 million if necessary.

Quick Facts

Specialty:	Multispecialty/Primary Care
CEO:	Charles G. Berg
Headquarters:	Norwalk, CT

Integrated Medical Network, Inc.

Integrated Medical Network, Inc., was formed for the purpose of operating a physician management company focusing primarily on orthopedics. IMN's strategy is to lead the consolidation taking place in the health care industry by creating networks of orthopedic surgeons, initially in Atlanta and other selected markets. IMN began operating its networks in the fall of 1996 with its founding affiliated physicians owning a controlling interest in the Company.

Quick Facts

Specialty:	Orthopedics
CEO:	James B. Cosgrove
Headquarters:	Atlanta, GA

Kelson Physician Partners, Inc.

Kelson Physician Partners, Inc. (formerly Prime Health), is a privately held pediatric practice management company based out of Bloomfield, Connecticut. Skip Creasey, CEO and President, established Kelson with physicians and managed care executives in 1994 to provide management expertise and investment capital for pediatric groups across the nation. Kelson has received financing from Marquette Venture Partners LP (Deerfield, IL), MVP Affiliates Fund (Boston, MA), and InterWest Partners (Menlo Park, CA).

6/19/97—Kelson has announced the intent to affiliate with Pediatric Associates of Wellesley, Inc., a pediatric practice in the Boston area.

5/29/97—Kelson formed a long-term partnership agreement with Tenafly Pediatrics, P.A., a leading pediatrics group in northern New Jersey.

9/06/96—Kelson entered a long-term partnership with Pediatric Associates, a 32-physician group practice in Hollywood, CA.

Quick Facts

Specialty:	Pediatrics
Chairman:	Skip Creasey
Headquarters:	Bloomfield, CT

MedFirst HealthCare, Inc.

MedFirst couples the latest in electronic connectivity with managed care networking and practice services. MedFirst focuses on solo and small group physicians, community hospitals, and local ancillary vendors who act as the hubs of its integrated system. MedFirst creates joint ventures with local providers to take advantage of capitated managed care opportunities, while offering them services such as billing and collection and employee leasing. Joint venture participants are electronically linked, maximizing economies of scale and reducing duplication of services while improving patient care and medical outcomes. MedFirst has joint ventures in the Midwest and on the East Coast with annual revenue of more than $100 million.

5/1/97—Primus Healthcare and MedFirst Healthcare have formed a joint venture, MSO South Florida. Through the joint venture, MedFirst will provide Primus with managed care and physician support services as well as access to existing patient care contracts.

Quick Facts

Specialty:	Multispecialty/Primary Care
Chairman:	Thomas S. Griffin, Jr, MD
Headquarters:	Culver City, CA

Physicians Quality Care, Inc.

Physicians Quality Care, Inc., provides practice management services for multispecialty medical practice groups. Its objective is to establish networks of primary and specialty care physicians and related diagnostic and therapeutic support services which can provide comprehensive health care services in targeted geographic areas. In June 1997, the company secured $100 million in capital from Bain Capital Inc. (Boston, MA), Goldman, Sachs and Co. (New York, NY), and ABS Capital Partners PC (Baltimore, MD—an investment fund associated with Alex. Brown & Sons). Physicians Quality Care manages 176 physicians in New England and the Mid-Atlantic states, and CEO Jerilyn Asher expects 1997 revenues to top $75 million. In April 1997 the company filed a shelf registration to enable it to use stock in its practice acquisitions and may go public within the next 12 months, depending on market conditions. Physicians currently own a controlling interest in PQC, holding seven of 11 of the seats on the firm's board.

Quick Facts

Specialty:	Multispecialty/Primary Care
CEO:	Jerilyn Asher
Headquarters:	Waltham, MA

Sedona Healthcare Group, Inc.

Sedona Healthcare Group, Inc., is focused on developing new networks of primary care physician practices in second- and third-tier cities, rural areas, and high-growth markets. The company currently owns 18 practice sites in Nevada, Arizona, Florida, Maryland, Virginia, and Indiana, which include a total of 30 physicians and mid-level providers. Sedona expects to add approximately 30 additional practices by the end of 1997. Also, Sedona provides management services to non-Sedona-owned physicians and plans to sign similar management agreements with an additional 120 to 140 doctors by the end of 1997. Sedona has received over $18 million from nine venture capital firms.

Quick Facts

Specialty:	Primary Care
CEO:	David Joyce
Headquarters:	Chapel Hill, NC

UniPhy HealthCare

UniPhy was founded in 1996 by Richard Francis, former senior vice president of development for HealthTrust. The Company currently manages over 250 physicians in four states as well as an IPA in Tennessee. Its objective is to provide resources and capital to local markets to build physician-directed delivery systems that are primary care oriented. Approximately $20 million of capital has been committed by Pacific Venture of Los Angeles, CA; Alex. Brown & Sons, and OrNda HealthCorp (OrNda was acquired by Tenet Healthcare in January 1997).

Quick Facts

Specialty:	Multispecialty/Primary Care
CEO:	Richard Francis, Jr
Headquarters:	Nashville, TN